Prevention Program
Development and Evaluation

In my experience it takes considerable dedication to work in the field of prevention. It's often an uncertain enterprise, as this question underscores: How can you tell if you've actually prevented something from occurring? So you have to be "true to your school," the school of prevention, that is.

Certainly dedication to prevention is required by practitioners, but teachers, scholars, and researchers all need a healthy dose of it, too. All of us are swimming against some strong tides—and making progress, too, as we seek to find verifiable ways to lessen new cases of human suffering and to promote healthy functioning.

Therefore, I dedicate Prevention Program Development and Evaluation *to all of you who have been involved, and to those who are joining the prevention effort. Keep the faith, be true to your school, and take encouragement from Matthew Arnold's 1866 poem "Thyrsis":*

Why faintest thou!

I wander'd till I died.

Roam on!

The light we sought

Is shining still. (Lancashire, 2008)

Prevention Program Development and Evaluation

An Incidence Reduction, Culturally Relevant Approach

Robert K. Conyne

University of Cincinnati

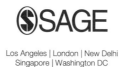

Los Angeles | London | New Delhi
Singapore | Washington DC

For information:

SAGE Publications, Inc.
2455 Teller Road
Thousand Oaks, California 91320
E-mail: order@sagepub.com

SAGE Publications India Pvt. Ltd.
B 1/I 1 Mohan Cooperative
    Industrial Area
Mathura Road, New Delhi 110 044
India

SAGE Publications Ltd.
1 Oliver's Yard
55 City Road
London EC1Y 1SP
United Kingdom

SAGE Publications Asia-Pacific Pte. Ltd.
33 Pekin Street #02-01
Far East Square
Singapore 048763

Printed in the United States of America.

Library of Congress Cataloging-in-Publication Data

Conyne, Robert K.
Prevention program development and evaluation: An incidence reduction, culturally relevant approach/Robert K. Conyne.
    p. cm.
Includes bibliographical references and index.
ISBN 978-1-4129-6679-5 (cloth)
ISBN 978-1-4129-6680-1 (pbk.)
    1. Preventive health services. I. Title.

RA425.C776 2010
614.4′4—dc22   2008055507

Printed on acid-free paper.

09   10   11   12   13   10 9 8 7 6 5 4 3 2 1

Acquiring Editor:	Kassie Graves
Editorial Assistant:	Veronica Novak
Production Editor:	Sarah K. Quesenberry
Copy Editor:	Teresa Wilson
Proofreader:	Jenifer Kooiman
Indexer:	Sheila Bodell
Typesetter:	C&M Digitals (P) Ltd.
Cover Designer:	Janet Foulger
Marketing Manager:	Carmel Schrire

Contents

List of Tables, Figures, and Learning Exercises

Tables

Figures

Learning Exercises

Preface

"Stayin' Alive," the Bee Gees' huge disco hit of 1977 (before the time of many of you!), can save lives due to its catchy tune and 103 beats per minute, the latter being perfectly in sync with the proper performance of chest compressions in cardiopulmonary resuscitation (CPR). A study reported at the annual meeting of the American College of Emergency Physicians by Dr. David Matlock of the University of Illinois College of Medicine at Peoria indicated that medical students and physicians who were trained in CPR while listening to the tune were able to maintain the proper CPR rhythm and also were able to reproduce it accurately weeks later. This finding is important because correctly delivered CPR can triple survival rates for cardiac arrest (Layton, 2008).

The proper delivery of CPR is a simple, but powerful, example of a prevention strategy. Indeed, prevention is coming to be understood as a necessity in physical health, mental health, and education. Note the following injunction, which concluded a newspaper article about the rise of suicides among middle-aged whites, particularly women, in the United States (Crane, 2008): "One thing on which the experts agree: *The study should prompt more prevention efforts* [italics added]."

In addition to becoming an essential ingredient in contemporary education and mental health, prevention is very much an everyday experience. Accumulating research attests that our mothers and everyday proverbs have been right all along— cautioning us to "look before we leap," "save for a rainy day," and "be prepared."

Applied to mental health, we understand the maxim that "an ounce of prevention is worth a pound of cure." Attending to both person-centered and system-centered programs can help people reduce the impact of stressors in their lives while using their strengths to build a better future. This approach can help them avoid dysfunction and reduce the costs of treatment. Yet too many helping professionals know neither how to teach prevention nor how to deliver it.

The minimal presence of prevention training in most academic programs continues to contribute to this deficit although, on the positive side of the ledger, the numbers of programs now offering prevention training show signs of increasing (Conyne, Newmeyer, Kenny, Romano, & Matthews, 2008). Drawing from the transtheoretical stages of change model (Prochaska & DiClemente, 2005), Adams (2008) suggested that prevention in counseling psychology may be moving from a contemplation stage (thinking about applying prevention) to the preparation stage, where people are beginning to incorporate it into practice and training. If so, then hooray, it's sure been a long time coming (Conyne, 2000)! Although it is encouraging that movement is occurring, plenty of space exists for implementing and maintaining prevention.

Certainly, one of the ways that prevention can be practiced lies within treatment approaches. In fact, a cogent argument can be launched that a major purpose of treatment (e.g., individual psychotherapy or counseling) is for clients to learn how to prevent reoccurrence of the problems (and of related concerns) that brought them to seek professional help in the first place. From this perspective, all treatment includes prevention, without dichotomy. I subscribe to that viewpoint. As I've pointed out previously,

> It is now possible to think and act in terms of viewing prevention and treatment along the same helping dimension, viewing them as collaborative partners, not as rivals. This is a far healthier position and is more apt to support both prevention and remediation. (Conyne, 2004, p. xv)

At the same time, though, prevention can be approached outside of treatment, as an end in its own right. Programs that are focused on prevention can be developed and delivered in an effort to forestall the emergence of new problems. This approach garners the attention of this book. Here, we are concerned with prevention programs—in and of themselves—and how to create them.

From that perspective, then, it can be noted that even as prevention is beginning to gain increased acceptability, it continues to lag behind problem remediation approaches. Uncertainties in how to develop and evaluate prevention programs— indeed, as I have said, the very subject of this book—are major factors in holding back prevention. Students and practitioners are left with the question: How do we "do prevention"?

Prevention Program Development and Evaluation: An Incidence Reduction, Culturally Relevant Approach seeks to address this problem. It is intended to provide direction for instructors, trainers, students, and practitioners in how to design and evaluate effective preventive interventions in mental health, education, and community settings by giving specific attention to the reduction of incidence (reducing new cases of a disorder), while giving credence to processes of collaboration, participation, and cultural relevance. Training workshops I conduct on prevention in mental health (both in the United States and abroad), the publication of new resources in prevention, accumulating evidence-based practice, and the increasing profile now given to prevention in counseling psychology (e.g., through the Prevention Section of the Society of Counseling Psychology) and other fields all suggest to me that interest and increasing importance are being placed on prevention as a concept and as a practice.

The rationale for this book is that program development and evaluation needs to be yoked more closely to prevention in order for prevention programs to become more frequently provided. This connection also will help prepare students and trainees to become more adept at prevention.

In this book, I attempt to describe how to develop and evaluate prevention programs and interventions guided by an incidence-reduction conceptual framework that was first suggested by Albee, which I have adapted over time (see Conyne & Newmeyer, 2008; Conyne, Newmeyer, & Kitchens, 2007). Although the book describes the entire program development and evaluation sequence, the purpose is to highlight it with regard to prevention programs.

Defining the problem identification step within program development and evaluation from the incidence reduction perspective of prevention commands the lion's share of attention. In addition, the incidence reduction lens is sharpened by incorporating processes of community, collaboration, and cultural relevance. I have successfully used this approach in teaching prevention and in training workshops, which both students and practitioners have found to be beneficial.

As implied above, many forces are serving to open up the teaching and practice of prevention. These include multicultural counseling and diversity, positive psychology, ecological approaches to counseling, group work, social justice, and culturally relevant practice. This expansion will continue noticeably, I believe. Why? Prevention and how to do it will become more mainstream as awareness builds that remediation is but one important approach to mental health and educational delivery and it needs to be complemented by other approaches. We are learning that in addition to the important and necessary work of helping people who already are dealing with problems, we also must figure out how to reach people "before the fact" in ways that are empirically sound and responsive to cultural characteristics. This is the essence of prevention.

Courses at both the undergraduate and graduate levels are being expanded to include prevention. When the curriculum can handle it, specialized courses are appearing that demand specialized texts. Otherwise, infusion occurs across existing courses, and prevention resources are included as supplements.

Some excellent (but few in number) sources exist in the area of prevention, including the examples that follow. Stellar prevention programs were identified and described in an American Psychological Association publication, *14 Ounces of Prevention* (Price, Cowen, Lorion, & Ramos-McKay, 1988). The forthcoming edited volume, *Realizing Social Justice: The Challenge of Preventive Interventions,* edited by Kenny, Horne, Orpinas, and Reese (2009), effectively examines how prevention connects with social justice. Major contributions have appeared in issues of *The Counseling Psychologist:* Romano and Hage (2000) discussed the relationship between prevention and counseling psychology; prevention guidelines were suggested (Hage et al., 2007); and culturally relevant prevention was considered by Reese and Vera (2007). A future special issue of the *Journal of Primary Prevention,* cited above, will feature methods of teaching primary prevention (O'Neil & Britner, in press).

Reviewers suggested that I comment specifically on how this new text differs from my 2004 text, *Preventive Counseling* (which abridged my original 1987 text). For years, these other texts were the only ones available to address prevention within counseling and counseling psychology. I intended them to "open the door" to prevention for counselors, to introduce them to its concepts and basic strategies. As such, these texts were basic primers in the field and, I think, crossed a new threshold. This new text very clearly builds on them while focusing on the essential process of program development in prevention. As I've pointed out earlier in this preface, *how to plan and evaluate* prevention programs now needs to be addressed, and that is what I have sought to do in this text. Providing an expansive and concrete way to apply incidence reduction within planning is an innovation that should advance prevention practice. In addition, I've incorporated the newest material available, particularly sources dedicated to cultural sensitivity and relevance, and to social justice.

Actually, the publication of a new book is no unique or special event anymore when you realize that today—meaning on *this* day, as every day—more than 3,000 books will be published (The Fischbowl, 2007)! Even so, at least book authors think their books are distinctive, as I confess I do.

I wrote this book for five types of courses: (a) human service courses at the undergraduate level; (b) existing prevention courses or courses in program development and evaluation; (c) introductory courses in graduate fields of helping, for example, Theories of Counseling, where this book could serve as a supplement; (d) practice-stage courses centered around practicum and internship, where students are providing supervised service; and (e) doctoral seminars. Beyond academic courses, due to its practical focus, this book will be of value to the large number of practicing counselors, psychologists, social workers, and others who are offering prevention programming without benefit of specific training.

Prevention Program Development and Evaluation addresses another key step for implementing prevention. Linking theory with practice, I have tried to show some of the nuts and bolts involved with converting the magnificent goal of prevention—which now enjoys considerable supportive research—to its execution within training programs and by helpers in the field.

The book contains a number of instructional resources and learning aids. Seven lighthearted figures are included to buoy readers as they move through the book. Each chapter is introduced by an overview, includes learning exercises (25 in all), and ends with a summary. Interspersed are five explanatory tables that summarize essential aspects of the overall prevention program development and evaluation process.

To make learning come increasingly alive, I strongly encourage readers in Chapter 7 to select their own prevention topic that they can work with as they proceed through Chapters 7–9; better yet, I suggest they form a team. Periodic process checks are presented as learning exercises to help a team assess its important work. The final chapter in this book provides readers with opportunities to apply their prevention analytical skills as they examine program descriptions against evaluative criteria.

The book concludes with an extensive and comprehensive set of classic and contemporary references in the prevention and program development fields and eight appendices that will be useful in applying information contained throughout the text. I have found in teaching and training that these kinds of organizers, exercises, resources, and summaries sensitize learners to what makes for good prevention programs.

I hope that this book will enable readers to climb another rung on the prevention ladder. Increased knowledge and skill in program development will enable personnel to launch prevention programs more frequently and effectively in mental health, educational, and community settings—thus contributing more fully to reducing the scope of social problems and to improving human satisfaction and fulfillment.

Acknowledgments

For decades I taught two specialized courses that I developed—preventive counseling, and program development and evaluation (this course with Lynn Rapin)—that students said should be linked together because they were so mutually reinforcing.

The present book attempts to provide that linkage. It is intended to serve as a guide for those interested in developing and evaluating prevention programs.

As with any book, many people are to be credited (but only I can take any blame). Early collaboration with Doug Lamb, Neal Gamsky, Jim Clack, Lynn Rapin, Betty Rademacher, Don Cochran, Fran LaFave, Bob Silver, Betty Harding (dec.), and other terrific professional staff and the paraprofessional student advisors at the Illinois State University (ISU) Student Counseling Service in the 1970s provided a dynamic crucible for developing campus-based preventive interventions, such as the environmental assessment project. In ISU's Counselor Education Program I first developed a fledgling preventive counseling elective course in 1975. The belief directing this course was, and remains, that counselors, psychologists, social workers, and other helpers need to function first as "preventionists," and that prevention should infuse all interventions. The basic structure of the course has been carried forward ever since, both at ISU and for 25 years in the Counseling Program at the University of Cincinnati (UC), where it moved from special topic, to elective, to required status—incorporating many twists and turns as research, training, and practice evolved. Also at ISU, Lynn and I developed the foundation for our program development and evaluation course, which was used there within counseling service consultation and training sessions. That course, too, later became a staple of the UC Counseling Program, and its contents formed the center of many consultation projects either of us assumed.

None of this academic activity would have been possible without the tolerance and support of my fellow faculty at both institutions, who fortunately gave me the benefit of the doubt to keep moving ahead. For instance, Ray Eiben (dec.) at ISU (in the middle 1970s) and Geof Yager at UC (early 1980s) first supported the initial special topics versions of the preventive counseling course in their respective Counseling Programs—in both cases, I think, wondering why they should do that—actions that were instrumental in allowing the course to develop, take hold, and then flourish. Thanks to them and to all of my colleagues at both institutions.

Scores and scores of students who took the preventive counseling course were my enthusiastic critics, always pushing me to become clearer, and they also were my collaborators all along the way; for instance, the preventive checklist contained in this book expanded after every class offering due to specific input from these students. A former UC counseling student, Mark Newmeyer, graciously volunteered to comment on a portion of this book manuscript; I thank him for his feedback and for assisting me several times in teaching both the preventive counseling and the program development and evaluation courses. Likewise, I thank Jeri Crowell and Gail Kiley, two other former UC Counseling Program students, for the multiple times they volunteered to assist me in teaching those courses. And I am especially pleased and thankful for the creative contribution of my brother, John Conyne, for his cartoons. I owe them all my gratitude.

My acquisitions editor at SAGE, Kassie Graves, stretching back to my book *Failures in Group Work,* deserves singular appreciation for her wisdom and her support of my work. The full range of SAGE staff also have been invaluable in producing this book, including Veronica Novak (editorial assistant), Sarah Quesenberry (production editor), and Teresa Wilson (copy editor). The observations and recommendations made by reviewers of this book, all prevention experts themselves and fellow travelers in the "prevention mission," were comprehensive and insightful, and I want to acknowledge each of them: Andy Horne, Mary Lee Nelson, James O'Neil, John Romano, Paul Richard Smokowski, Elizabeth Vera, and Michael Waldo. The Prevention Section of the American Psychological Association's Society of Counseling Psychology (similar to the American College Personnel Association Commission VII's prevention task force and the APA Division 17 Prevention Interest Group of the 1970s) provides a fount of innovative ideas and a wonderful sense of mutual support, and it has been an honor for me to be involved. The late Bob Toal first exposed me to community psychology at Purdue University during my doctoral program, for which I am ever grateful. Rudy Moos from Stanford was a strong early influence from afar on my thinking about social ecology in prevention, as were Jim Banning and Jim Hurst in the area of campus ecology. Rick Price, with whom I completed a year (years ago) as a postdoctoral scholar in community psychology at the University of Michigan, taught me much about prevention's value, strategies, and research, and I thank him for his mentorship.

And finally my family deserves special mention for allowing me the time to stare at my computer screen attempting to untangle my cobwebbed thoughts by writing—to my wife and colleague, Lynn; my daughter, Suzanne; my son, Zack; and our dog, Lucy (who always lies at my feet as I plod along, providing an unquestioned supportive foundation)—thank you!

SECTION I

Prevention Foundation

We exist in a rapidly evolving world. One aspect of this constant and fast change involves the myriad applications of technology that are available and constantly being both revised and innovated. The Web site www.youtube.com provides an example of one contemporary mode of accessing and contributing to knowledge and experience. So, let us start our focus on prevention by drawing from a video contained on that medium called "The Wisdom of Prevention" by John Fung (2008), who is an herbalist. He indicates in the video that prevention is the foundation of Chinese medicine and it first was discussed in 300 BC in *The Book of the Interior,* or *Nei Jing.* He presents a quotation from that source that underlines the importance of prevention: "The superior healer is one who can successfully check diseases before they develop." Fung goes on to say that prevention involves a lifestyle that is enjoyable and sensible, includes a regularity of moderate practices, is not costly, and is broadly applied.

Fung's notion of prevention represents an important perspective, which I call "everyday prevention" (Conyne, 2004) and discuss in the following chapter. Lifestyle accounts for 50%–80% of healthy and unhealthy functioning. Therefore, personal choice and responsibility can contribute strong preventive effects. Personal habits, skills, and dispositions all play critical roles in maintaining our well-being and in protecting us from risk. Examples include what we eat and drink, how much we exercise, and our coping skills for managing stress and relating to others.

However, we live within ongoing contexts that are themselves influential. Settings, such as work and community, and differing levels of environments ranging from close relationships to distant forces such as economic conditions in Japan dynamically interact to affect us in both obvious and subtle ways. An important aspect of prevention, then, is that which is beyond self-responsibility but is centered on environmental and systemic factors.

In every case, the Latin meaning of prevention—"to come before"—is central.

CHAPTER 1

Prevention in Everyday Life

The Basic Logic of Prevention

As a teenager I used to watch a weekly television show called "The Naked City." Every show concluded with the same voiceover: "There are 8 million stories in the Naked City. This has been one of them" (Tatara, 2008).

I thought of that tagline when considering prevention because it seems that there are at least 8 million physical health, mental health, and education problems—in the naked city, or otherwise—that press upon all of us. Of course, we cannot correct all of them, certainly not by restricting our efforts to individual remediation, and besides, there are far too few trained helpers available. That's where prevention comes in. Presented next is information related to just one broad set of problems facing society today—violence.

According to the U.S. Office of Juvenile Justice and Delinquency Prevention (American Psychological Association Commission on Violence and Youth, 1996), a 40% increase in murders, robberies, rapes, and assaults was reported to law enforcement agencies between 1985 and 1994, with youth accounting for 26% of that increase in violence. The related prevention question is: How can these negative outcomes be averted? Holding off new problems from developing is the central thesis of prevention. Correcting the effects of already existing problems— although important and necessary to do—is the opposite of prevention, and reliance on it is inevitably a losing game. It cannot be mentioned too often that there are many more problems existing and developing every day than there are helpers to address them, especially if a 1:1 remedial model is relied upon (Albee, 1985; Conyne, 2004; Romano & Hage, 2000). Just as the little Dutch boy cannot forever hold off the building waters that eventually will burst through the dam, failing to use prevention ultimately is too little, too late.

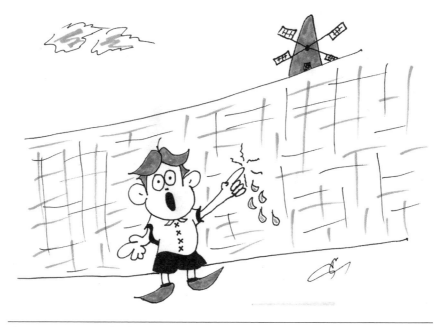

Figure 1.1   Hey! Why didn't we plug this hole?

Source: © John Conyne.

Of course, we could just as easily substitute other negative conditions and outcomes for violence and the exact same logic would apply—obesity, school dropouts, depression, suicide, cancer, and legions more. Can these negative outcomes be prevented, or the number of new cases reduced?

Returning to the violence example, the following preventive mind-set is essential:

Rather than waiting until violence has been learned and practiced and then devoting increased resources to hiring policemen, building more prisons, and sentencing three-time offenders to life imprisonment, it would be more effective to redirect the resources to early violence prevention programs, particularly for young children and preadolescents. (http://www.apa.org/ppo/issues/pbviolence.html)

There is much essential logic contained in the quotation presented above. It happens to be focused on the issue of violence, which is a vital concern in our communities and around the world. Boiled down to its basic elements, the logic is:

Before-the-fact programs and everyday best practices can prevent negative conditions and outcomes from occurring or, at the least, lessen their duration and severity while they build and broaden competencies.

Everyday Prevention: We Always Knew That Mom Was (Almost Always) Right

Attending to before-the-fact programs characterizes prevention. There is absolutely nothing mysterious or magical about the logic undergirding this approach. In fact, it is the warp and woof of many maternal injunctions and common life proverbs.

Craik (1991) observed that "lives are lived day by day, one day at a time, from day to day, day after day, day in and day out. Lives as we experience them are inherently quotidian" (p. 1). James Joyce (1961), in *Ulysses,* creatively exhausted this concept as he wrote in expansive detail about an ordinary day (June 16, 1904) in the life of the main character, Leopold Bloom, as he moves through Dublin. Everyday prevention is a phrase that captures ordinary, day-by-day occurrences that can serve to nurture and support people. As such, it recognizes the positive aspects of Craik's quotidian.

In some ways, everyday prevention represents the obverse of the multicultural concept of racial "microaggressions" (D. W. Sue et al., 2008) in everyday life. These are defined as "brief and commonplace verbal, behavioral, and environmental indignities, whether intentional or unintentional, that communicate hostile, derogatory, or negative racial slights and insults to the target person or group" (D. W. Sue et al., 2007, p. 273).

Conversely, in everyday prevention, we look for what might be termed "microbuffers"—the smaller, everyday attitudes, behaviors, activities, and environmental cues that, when observed or practiced on a daily basis, can contribute to and support positive mental health while arresting adverse effects. (Note: I owe this conceptual tie of everyday prevention to microaggressions to an observation made by Maureen Kenny of the Prevention Section of the Society of Counseling Psychology.) Taking a lead from D. W. Sue (2003), it would be useful to investigate the role that coping skills and microbuffers might play in counteracting microaggressions.

For instance, you may have been instructed while growing up to attend to these everyday aphorisms:

"An ounce of prevention is worth a pound of cure" (value of prevention)

"Look before you leap" and "Stop, look, and listen" (be observant)

"Only *you* can prevent forest fires" (take personal responsibility)

"An apple a day keeps the doctor away" (practice good nutrition)

"Be prepared" (be ready for life events)

"Save for a rainy day" (defer gratification)

"Do unto others as you would have them do unto you" (be respectful)

No doubt you can think of other maxims that serve a similar purpose of providing some useful everyday life guidance and, if followed, might reduce problems and allow for a happier life ("Don't go near the water until you learn how to swim" comes to mind). They represent examples of what I have called "everyday prevention" (Conyne, 2004), or how we can build into our daily lives good practices that are associated with healthy living.

Everyday prevention refers to "people enacting daily life best practices in context to optimize functioning and avert significant problems" (Conyne, 2004, p. 34).

Examples of significant problems to be avoided—indeed, the top 10 major public health issues in the United States—include (U.S. Department of Health and Human Services [U.S. DHHS], 2000): physical inactivity, overweight and obesity, tobacco use, substance use, irresponsible sexual activity, mental unhealthiness, injury and violence, environmental pollution, lack of immunization, and insufficient and lack of ready access to health care. The practice of everyday prevention by increasing numbers of citizens can contribute to reducing the frequency and intensity of these and other health issues.

The Ruby and Oren Principle

Following is an everyday prevention story that I have told in previous sources (e.g., Conyne, 2004), as I suppose one can with a principle. Thirty years ago my wife, Lynn Rapin, and I lived next door to a wonderful couple in their late 80s, named Ruby and Oren. We became aware that every Saturday afternoon they met with friends to play cards. Sometimes this meant traveling several miles over wintry roads to a hosting couple's home. Not being a card player, I had always wondered what could possibly be so engaging about this activity—especially when Oren told me one day that he and Ruby had to miss "just our third gathering in 35 years" due to icy road conditions! This tipped me over the edge; I couldn't hold back my amazement any longer. So I asked Oren what kept this card-playing gathering going over all those years? He thought for a moment, and then said that it wasn't really about card playing; rather, it was that gathering together to play cards every week gave them the excuse to get together with friends, to laugh and carp about things, to catch up on events in each other's lives, and to feel good in each other's company. I think this is such a powerful story about the value of social support and active engagement—or what Eric Erickson (1986) termed "vital involvement"—that it can be viewed as an everyday prevention best practice. I later dubbed it the "Ruby and Oren Principle" (Conyne, 2004, pp. 34–35).

The Case of Dental Flossing

Regular dental care provides a concrete illustration of everyday prevention practice. Key aspects include dental flossing (discussed below) and the initiative to make a dental checkup a prerequisite for school enrollment. Tooth decay and gum disease are major problems. In Kentucky, for example, 40% of adults over age 65 have had all their teeth extracted, and in Ohio the percentage is 25. Across the nation pediatric dental associations report a significant increase in childhood dental cavities, even in baby teeth. Consequences of dental problems are not restricted to the teeth, according to the American Academy of Pediatric Dentistry. In addition, cavities and gum disease can negatively affect children's school performance, self-esteem, and social relationships. For adults, poor dental health adds to improper nutrition, inflammation, and elevated risk for cardiovascular and other diseases ("Editorial: An Early Date," 2008).

Dental flossing is a practical, everyday activity that can help avert oral hygiene woes. But it also can do more than that. Bacteria that cause gum disease and loss of teeth may also contribute to heart disease, stroke, and other diseases (American Academy of Periodontology, 2005). Therefore, there are lots of reasons to floss.

If you don't floss (that is, don't exercise this kind of good preventive care), you might turn out like poor Charlie below.

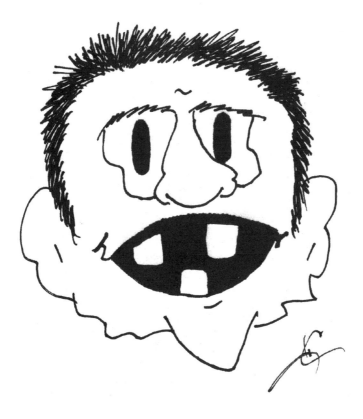

Figure 1.2 Charlie didn't take time to floss.

Source: © John Conyne.

I use flossing to concretely demonstrate how a simple but important everyday prevention act can occur.

On the first day of my prevention course, I typically ask students to close their eyes and to raise their hand if they floss their teeth regularly (I don't want to invade personal privacy and embarrass anyone). I count the hands and report the results. Then I proceed to discuss dental flossing and its preventive values while I— intentionally violating any form of good etiquette, taste, and decorum—proceed to floss my teeth (briefly) in front of them. Yes, I know this is gross. But they do not forget the lesson, either, and this demonstration helps to create a basic understanding of how prevention can occur. The issue becomes, "What is the equivalent of dental floss in mental health?" or its corollary, "Is there a 'mental floss,' and how can it be created and delivered?" Some mental health equivalents include careful listening, conveying empathy, playing games with friends (remember Ruby and Oren), meditating daily, communing with nature, exercising, volunteering, and participating actively in organizations and community life. Again, active engagement, or vital involvement, runs through these activities. What others can you think of? That is the question I ask students.

I close this class segment by reporting two dental stories. The first is from my dentist. While working on my teeth, he told me that none of his five children had chosen to follow in his footsteps to eventually take over the family business because they believed that the emphasis on prevention in dental practice might ultimately eliminate the need for dentists because people would learn how to avoid dental problems. Sometimes students and practitioners have raised this very issue with me, too, wondering if there would be anything left for counselors to do if prevention were really to become successful. Do not fear, I say with confidence, there will always be enough psychological and emotional problems to go around! The second story is from a friend of mine who has been practicing dentistry for 35 years. When trying to influence his patients to floss daily, he says he often uses a light touch, in this case, a dental joke. He advises them, "Well, flossing isn't such a big thing—just floss the teeth you want to keep" (Caddoo, 2000).

A core process involved in everyday prevention is positive engagement, as I have mentioned. Those people who are actively involved in constructive activities on a regular basis seem to enjoy a built-in immunity to life's slings and arrows. Not that they will be able to totally avoid major life problems, but they will be better able to resist onslaughts, to find value and meaning in their lives, and to continue moving ahead.

Prevention Is in the News and All Around Us

The popular media is full of prevention-related stories, some mostly accurate, others mostly the reverse. You have to be careful. But to find them, all you have to do is to look intentionally. On the second day of class I ask students in my prevention course to do just that, and to bring to class prevention-oriented stories they discover. Please note that I intentionally instruct the students not to work too hard to discover these items. That instruction is quite contrary to typical expectations for the prevention course and is usually welcomed. Attending to popular media coverage is in addition to reading the assigned professional literature for the course, which is substantial (students marvel, not always glowingly!).

I tell them that the topics they find in everyday sources could include such disparate everyday prevention activities as the already-familiar tooth flossing, car maintenance, psychological benefits of playing Wii, getting sufficient sleep, national defense, and the value of friendship. Moreover, they might come across stories associated with mental health and education prevention programs, such as in the areas of bullying, obesity, dropouts, addictions, positive psychology, and stress.

For the most part, the items come from the local newspaper, radio, television channels, or the Internet. In fact, success in finding prevention news items from local sources illustrates the very point I am trying to make in this exercise: *If we focus our attention, we will find that prevention is all around us, not some esoteric, highly specialized approach.*

Recently I engaged in this activity by attending to the local media for "prevention news." Nearly every day I came across viable items, such as preventive tips for managing stress, provided on the John Tesh (2008) radio show, "Intelligence for Your Life" (see also www.tesh.com). You might try attending to popular media for prevention-oriented messages yourself for a period of time and note what you find.

For instance, talk about timing, just as I was writing the preceding sentence, I received an e-mail from the National Youth Anti-Drug Media Campaign (2008) about how the family medicine cabinet can serve as an unintended source for teenage illicit drug use. How? Prescribed and over-the-counter drugs for parents kept in medicine cabinets (or sometimes on bathroom or kitchen counters) are all-too-readily accessible for abuse by others. An everyday prevention act in this domain is to safeguard these medications, set clear rules for teens, be a good role model in how you use and take care of medicines, and properly dispose of old medicines. Incidentally, when I was out of town recently, my wife decided to clean out our bathroom cabinets. Alarmingly, she found and disposed of several expired prescribed medications.

Following are some other examples of stories that I came across first in the popular press, often from the local newspaper. If the story was local in scope, I went no further. If, however, it was reporting on a research study or intervention that was reported first in a scholarly source, I then went to the scholarly publication. Keeping in mind the caveat to be wary of the accuracy of research reported in the popular media, let's take a look at some examples.

In junior and senior high school I lived with my family in remote, small towns in frigid, forlorn, yet beautiful upstate New York, 3 miles from the Quebec, Canada, border. Our seventh-grade English teacher at Mooers Central School, Mrs. Ferns, decided that her 15 students—rubes that most of us were, with most not knowing of the existence of salad forks—sorely needed etiquette training. Over several class periods (seeming like a few years) she covered such everyday issues as how to greet another person, with which hand to hold a fork, and what clothes might be appropriate for which function. She taught us from George Washington's

(1971) *Rules of Civility and Decent Behaviour in Company and Conversation,* from the then-popular book by the singer Pat Boone (1958), *'Twixt Twelve and Twenty,* and from scenarios she seemed to have constructed on the spot. For instance, George Washington's *Rules* included 110 injunctions, such as Number 104: "It belongs to the Chiefest in Company to unfold his Napkin and fall to Meat first, But he ought then to Begin in time & to Dispatch with Dexterity that the Slowest may have time allowed him." A little ponderous and old fashioned, but I suppose worthy in intent, going through all 110 of these directives seemed a bit much to 13-year-olds from the boonies.

Looking back at it, though, it is clear to me that this was a kind of psycho-educational approach to prevention; that is, the prevention of embarrassment and social faux pas. Careers can be influenced by using proper etiquette. Mrs. Ferns apparently was ahead of her time. My daughter, Suzanne, who is now in her third year of study in a doctor of pharmacy program, tells me that students in her program participate in required etiquette training as part of their career preparation.

All this leads me to an item in today's newspaper (Mracek, 2008) containing a helpful preventive hint for proper table manners during business meals. Have you ever (as I have) sat down at a luncheon only to be uncertain about which bread plate and which drink glass is yours and which ones belong to those seated to your right and to your left? Here comes your preventive tip. Ms. Mracek advises us to (under the table so no one can notice) hold out both hands. (This works best, I discovered through practice, if you then tilt each hand 90 degrees.) Connect each index finger with its respective thumb to form a circle while holding the other three fingers of each hand out straight. If you have performed this exercise correctly, you should see that a small letter "b" is formed with the left hand and a "d" with the right. Respectively, these letters stand for **b**read and **d**rink. So now when you look at your dinner plate at formal functions, you will never be confused that your bread dish will be at the left and your drinking glass at the right of your plate—as long as you remember this bit of basic, everyday prevention advice. Although it's not necessarily psychological or emotional in scope, applying this tip can help to smooth social involvement and avoid errors, which sometimes can be costly. Now let's move to other kinds of examples of prevention being all around us in the news.

Health-information Web sites have become plentiful and, for many people, a frequent way to obtain information. A listing of the most popular ones was published by HealthDay news service (http://www.healthday.com). As of January 2008, there were 2,070 of these sites, compared with 1,047 in 2005. This increase reflects the mounting attention being given to health promotion and the thirst for information about it. As of February 9, 2008, the most popular sites, based on market share, were www.WebMD.com, www.MayoClinic.com, Yahoo! Health, MSN Health & Fitness, www.RightHealth.com, www.MedicineNet.com, www.ensuringsolutions.org, www .Drugs.com, Everyday Health, Revolution Health, and KidsHealth. This listing is not presented as an endorsement but, rather, to illustrate the sort of prevention-oriented information that is readily available today.

Here is an example from one of these sources, www.ensuringsolutions.org, a Web site from the George Washington University Medical Center. It is focused on alcohol problems and prevention and on possible related consequences of alcohol problems, such as diabetes and psychological dysfunction. Bruzzese (2008) describes a workplace approach for employers to consider using when suspecting an employee of excessive drinking. Addressing this problem early is important because alcohol problems account for millions of dollars in employer costs every year through lowered productivity, exploding health care costs, and a range of other serious negative health issues for the employee and her or his family. Abbreviated as AIM, the approach includes these steps: (a) Aim your message at the person directly, (b) Inform him or her of your observations, and (c) Motivate the person to seek help. The following interaction illustrates the AIM approach: "You know, you seem to be drinking more—how much are you drinking?" After a reply, this question might be followed by informing the employee that the amount and frequency he or she is drinking appears at work to be excessive. Finally, try to motivate the employee to seek help by expressing your concern and asking if she or he has thought about changing. Having ready referral sources available also is important.

Incidentally, similar early action is taking root now in an attempt to avert campus suicides and homicides (Peale, 2008). This proactive approach has developed since the Virginia Tech University rampage of April 16, 2007, modifying strict adherence to the 1974 Family Educational Rights and Privacy Act. Threat assessment groups (or their equivalent) have been formed on campuses to review records of students about whom a report of threatening behavior has been received. The information is shared among appropriate campus offices, and in some cases, these students are contacted and referred to the counseling center or, more rarely, to a local hospital for evaluation. In some cases, time-limited counseling sessions are mandated. Colleges and universities also have refined their capacity to immediately notify their constituencies of any emergency situation by using e-mails, text messages, and loudspeakers. And across campuses, students, professors, staff, and administrators have become more sensitized to the possibility of violent behavior occurring and to how to take appropriate action.

Now let us return to health information and practices. Aspirin is said to be an over-the-counter wonder drug, and it can have many medicinal benefits if used appropriately. You may recall the old joke where the doc can sound authoritative even while not having a clue about what's ailing the patient: "Take two aspirins and call me in the morning." Yet the appropriate use of aspirin has a solid track record, without serious side effects for most people, for treating or supplementing treatment of a wide range of common physical problems. In terms of prevention, you may have noticed, or in fact benefited from, the use of so-called "baby aspirin" (81 mg) in its role of lowering the risk of certain cardiac events. Found in a *Newsweek* magazine advertisement section on "Heart Health" is the following:

Aspirin has also been shown to prevent heart disease in men over 45 and women over 65 who don't have heart disease (what's called primary prevention), as well as preventing stroke in women under 65. In a meta-analysis of six primary

> prevention trials, researchers at the University of Alabama at Birmingham concluded that regular aspirin use decreases the risk of heart disease and non-fatal heart attacks. ("Heart Health," 2008, p. 8, Advertising Section)

Although it always is important to be skeptical of advertising material, in fact the evidence for safe and effective aspirin benefits in a heart-healthy lifestyle is generally accepted medically. Even my own family practice doctor at the University Medical Center, generally highly resistant to prescribing medication, asks me to take a daily 81-mg dose of aspirin as part of a heart-healthy approach. Back to the above quotation, it is interesting, too, for including the concept of primary prevention. Once-a-day, low-dosage aspirin is a convenient and cost-effective prevention strategy practiced by millions of Americans who are presently free from heart disease, as well as those with multiple risk factors like high blood pressure, family history of heart disease, or high cholesterol. (Note, however, that a recent study by Belch et al., 2008, reported that aspirin use did not prevent a first heart attack among participants who had diabetes or peripheral arterial disease). But not all who could potentially benefit are engaging in this preventive approach, such as African Americans and those with diabetes. As Goldberg (2008) points out, aspirin (or any other prevention strategy) will not work if it is not taken regularly.

Pregnancy and caffeine have also been receiving attention. Denise Grady of the *New York Times* summarized a recent study (Weng, Odouli, & Li, 2008) contained in the *American Journal of Obstetrics and Gynecology.* Researchers found that pregnant women drinking 200 mg of caffeine a day (the equivalent of a 10-ounce cup of coffee) may double their risks of miscarriage (Grady, 2008). Results of this study led the March of Dimes to plan on advising pregnant women, or those trying to conceive, to limit their daily caffeine intake to less than 200 mg.

How to dispense flu shots efficiently is a subject of much consideration. A simple but elegant prevention program was described by Daniel Yee of the Associated Press (2007). In this program, air travelers passing through some U.S. airport security checkpoints can receive a flu shot. Lee reported that this practice had been offered for a few years before passengers cleared security, but many were reluctant to take the shot for concern of being delayed during the security check, adding to the chance of missing their flight. Moving the service "airside," past security, helped to mitigate the anxiety about missing a flight while maintaining convenience. According to the newspaper account, 9,500 travelers had been vaccinated at O'Hare and Midway airports in Chicago alone prior to the onset of the 2007–2008 flu season.

A prevention program that currently is under development would create a mobile unit staffed and managed by the Cincinnati VA Medical Center (Wilkinson, 2007). This mobile health van would go to events that veterans are likely to attend, allowing them to complete enrollment paperwork and be initially screened for physical health, dental, and mental health issues. This service (which is in a fundraising phase) would make it unnecessary for vets to make two or more trips from their home to the VA Medical Center before ever receiving treatment.

Seeking to quickly improve the health status of male congregants, a pastor demanded in a Sunday sermon that all 900 male members of his congregation see a doctor within the next month (Welsh-Huggins, 2008). The pastor was reported to be shocked by the high rates of prostate cancer and diabetes suffered by black men and the low numbers of them receiving medical attention. Church deacons were made responsible to follow up on each member's progress. This preventive effort, noteworthy for its simplicity and directness, could make a positive difference in healthy functioning for the men who take advantage of it and sustain their involvement.

Another project that involved reminders (King et al., 2007) was conducted in the domain of physical exercise, an activity that many Americans find difficult to initiate and maintain. The study explored if a convenient, low-cost intervention might be effective in promoting consistent physical exercise. The study found that computer-generated phone call reminders were as effective as, and more efficient than, calls made by health educators to encourage participants to exercise weekly for 150 minutes ("Try It," 2008).

Lifestyle in relation to longevity is a subject of increasing attention. The Quest Network (2006) has identified "blue zones," a term used to refer to places where people live long lives. These locations where people seem to live longer than anywhere else are found in Loma Linda, California; Sardinia, Italy; and Okinawa, Japan (Buettner, 2008a). A fourth geographic area also has been identified, the Nicoya Peninsula of Costa Rica (Buettner, 2008b). Research of centenarians living in this region reveals everyday prevention lifestyle practices that seem to be powerfully associated with a lengthy, satisfying life.

These long-livers (a) have developed a strong sense of purpose, (b) drink hard water containing high calcium content, (c) maintain a focus on family, (d) eat a light dinner, (e) sustain social networks, (f) keep hard at work, (g) take in some "sensible" sun regularly, and (h) embrace a common history with strong spiritual traditions. For a fascinating look at one exemplar of long life in Nicoya, see the online video at www.aarpmagazine.org/lifestyle, which will introduce you to 101-year-old Panchita Castillo, who still rises at 4:00 a.m., chops wood, meets daily with friends and family, reveres life, and places her fate in a higher power.

A study from the University of Cambridge (Khaw et al., 2007) and summarized in the *Cincinnati Enquirer* on January 9, 2008 ("Good Habits Yield Longer Life"), tracked 20,000 people in the UK from 1993 to 1997. It found that an extra 14 years of life can be gained on average by not smoking, eating lots of fruits and vegetables, exercising regularly, and drinking alcohol moderately. Results also showed that the risk of death (particularly from cardiovascular disease) decreases as the number of positive health behaviors increases, suggesting that modest and achievable lifestyle changes could have a marked effect on the health of populations. These benefits were independent of social class or weight.

Speaking of weight, obesity in most developed countries is an epidemic. In the United States, England, and Australia, for example, more than half of adults are overweight or obese, with trend data showing a marked prevalence increase. In fact, youth today may be the first ever to live fewer years than their parents. Those who are obese are at heightened risk for disease and disability, including depression, diabetes, and heart disease (U.S. DHHS, 2001).

An editorial contained in the *Cincinnati Enquirer* ("Editorial: Following a New Path," 2008) supported the proposal made by President Pro Tem Katie Stine in the Kentucky Senate to require that any new state roads be constructed with walking and biking paths alongside them. Following is a quote from that editorial:

> As states and communities grapple with obesity and inactivity, they often realize too late that community design is a big part of the problem. A lack of sidewalks and bike lanes, congested traffic and a lack of destinations for walkers and bikers are obstacles to a healthy, active community. . . . We hope that legislators will get moving on an approach that will get citizens moving as well. (p. C-6)

Prevention news can be found easily regarding other topics beyond health, such as this next entry dealing with school dropouts. Larry Davis, a School and Families Empowerment (SAFE) agent for the Walton-Verona Independent Schools in northern Kentucky, keeps kids from dropping out. Over the last 9 years not one of the 1,500 students in grades P–12 has dropped out of school (Croyle, 2007). Davis said,

> I don't let parents or kids use the word "dropout" in my office. . . . Having no dropouts is a residual effect. I try to help students figure out their problems and help parents with their problems. If I can help get pressure off a kid, they'll probably graduate. (p. B-1)

Schooling affords a rich topic for prevention, indeed. In another example, the U.S. Department of Labor reports (see The Fischbowl, 2007) that one in four workers today has been with their present employer for less than 1 year, and one in two has been with their current employer for less than 5 years. In fact, in what might seem a startling forecast, the department estimates that today's students will have 10 to 14 jobs by their 38th birthday! What are the preventive implications for this sea change (one of many) in our society?

Accidental injuries are the subject of prevention. A study in *Injury Prevention* (Phelan, Khoury, Atherton, & Kahn, 2007) suggested that children of depressed mothers are more than twice as likely as other children to suffer injuries requiring medical attention (O'Farrell, 2007). These women are less likely to use child-occupant restraints, to have functioning smoke detectors in their homes, to clear up clutter, and to use the back-sleeping position for their infants compared with nondepressed mothers. Increased injuries occur in such situations. This study was said to be the first one to demonstrate a direct link between maternal depression and increased risk for childhood injury. The preventive implications are clear. If maternal depression can be diagnosed and treated early, then mothers are more likely to be able to learn and employ preventive strategies to eliminate injuries in their children.

Indeed, prevention is "all around us." The previous descriptions simply represent examples. If prevention is so commonplace, as the information extracted from popular media suggests, then what is its status in the helping professions? Here, prevention could be said to be only partially in place. The prevention zeitgeist has not yet made its way obviously within the helping professions.

LEARNING EXERCISE 1.1

Finding Everyday Prevention in Your World

Okay, now it's your turn. What is in your "everyday prevention" world? For the next week, take a good look at that world. Note especially information and images contained in the popular media.

Take notes of what you find that is linked with prevention. Return to this exercise box after you review your notes at week's end. What did you find? List five of the more interesting items below:

1. _____

2. _____

3. _____

4. _____

5. _____

Summarize what you learned from doing this exercise:

_____

_____

_____

Prevention in the Helping Fields

Like a freight train slowly inching up a long grade, prevention chugs along in the helping fields, making gradual gains. Although signs of progress are occurring, its rate needs to be revved up so that prevention can accelerate in psychology, counseling, social work, and the helping services.

To illustrate the situation, Romano and Hage (2000) in a "Call to Action" and Conyne (2000) in a proposed "Resolution" urged counseling psychology to accelerate its commitment to prevention through increased concrete actions in training, research, practice, and advocacy. Leadership in these areas is necessary to lower the barriers that inadvertently serve to keep the preventive profile low.

The barrier that is targeted in this book is that many professional helpers function without guidance about how to conduct prevention within the context of their role and function. This deficit is not their fault, of course. For the most part, practitioners were largely unexposed to prevention in their professional training. This situation is gradually improving, however, and optimistic signs are emerging.

For instance, the American Psychological Association (APA), whose overall purpose is "to advance psychology as a science and profession and as a means of promoting health, education, and human welfare" (American Psychological Association, 2008a), sponsors prevention programs as one of many methods to fulfill its purpose. Three brief examples from APA will be described next: (a) the Psychologically Healthy Workplaces Award program (American Psychological Association, 2008b), (b) cooperative program with the YMCA's Activate America campaign (Anderson, 2008), and (c) Adults and Children Together Against Violence (ACT) program (DeAngelis, 2008).

The Psychologically Healthy Workplaces Award (PHWA) program formally recognizes work settings that reduce job stress (which is estimated at costing U.S. employers $300 billion per year), while improving employee satisfaction, retention, and productivity. Qualifying organizations receive a special award that recognizes their commitment to programs and policies that enhance the health and well-being of their employees while fostering improved organizational productivity and performance. Five criteria are used to identify how effectively organizations support their employees' (a) involvement, (b) work-life balance, (c) growth and development, (d) health and safety, and (e) recognition. Employee productivity also is emphasized.

The PHWA program of the American Psychological Association is noteworthy for at least three reasons. The fact that a professional association would devote some of its time and resources to implement a procedure for recognizing work settings that demonstrate psychologically healthy environments is—at least in my mind—a credit to the association itself. Second, focusing on work organizations illustrates one aspect of a broad reach in prevention because these settings—in which millions of employees spend around one third of their waking hours every work week—are virtual petri dishes that can germinate both unhealthy and healthy processes and behaviors. Work organizations that promote healthy functioning in their employees, then, serve as preventive forces. Third, these winning programs have produced documentable gains in lowered stress, worker satisfaction, and higher productivity. These accomplishments are to be applauded. The fact that the evaluation models used may not allow these results to rise to the level demanded of empirically based interventions (see, especially, Chapters 3 and 6 of this book) suggests directions for growth.

In a second program, APA's Practice, Science, and Public Interest directorates along with its Division 42 (Independent Practice) are collaborating with the YMCA to tackle the obesity crisis in the United States. More than 60 million adults and 5 million youth in this country are obese, contributing to annual hospital costs for this condition that have increased three times over the previous two decades. As Norman Anderson, the APA's Chief Executive Officer, observes, the 2,617 YMCA settings reach huge numbers of young people, making them the largest child care provider in the nation. This extensive reach includes 20 million members spread across more than 8,500 communities and neighborhoods. Such a wide net makes the partnering of APA with that organization, which deals with lifestyle and behavioral issues involved with obesity, a natural fit. Educational workshops for parents on family connectedness, healthy eating, exercise, and other relevant areas will be presented by psychologists. In addition, policymakers will receive fact sheets and policy recommendations for the prevention of youth obesity. This promising prevention program is in the early stages of implementation.

In the third example, in 2000 the APA through its Violence Prevention Office launched a research-based primary prevention intervention, the Adults and Children Together Against Violence program. The ACT is intended to enhance positive parenting and to reduce maltreatment of children. This is an important area to address because, according to data from the Centers for Disease Control and Prevention (2005, cited by DeAngelis, 2008), the prevalence of child maltreatment is both high (e.g., 906,000 U.S. children have been identified as being maltreated, no doubt an underestimate) and potentially deadly (e.g., as reported in the data, 1,500 children died from maltreatment, including 36% from neglect, 28% from physical abuse, and 29% from multiple means). ACT is a basic, universal parenting program in which parents learn how to deal with anger, how children's developmental stages affect their behavior, the use of positive ways to discipline, and how to decrease the effect of media violence on children. This program has been evaluated through self-assessments and now is advancing to a national, three-site outcome study.

So, progress in providing prevention programs is occurring, which certainly is encouraging. However, to bring us back to the main point, creating and delivering preventive services remains a daunting challenge for too many practitioners. Frameworks, blueprints, and examples of how to design and deliver prevention programs are needed, as I have emphasized.

Before we consider how to do prevention, though, it is necessary to begin with a discussion of what prevention in mental health, education, and communities is. Although it is perhaps comforting to realize that prevention is commonplace in our culture and that our moms were right on this score after all—witness the aphorisms and news stories presented earlier—it will be useful first to consider prevention more deeply. The following chapter on the basic tenets of prevention begins with a brief excursion into some historical influences.

Summary

We come to prevention naturally. Whether through the homely bromides of our mothers or attributed to American heroes such as George Washington, we have inculcated advice for daily living. "Only YOU can prevent a forest fire," said Smokey the Bear, who is but one of these guides.

This chapter was meant to remind you that prevention is not some esoteric extra but it is part of the warp and woof of our everyday existence. It has also seeped into professional practice, training, and research. It is our responsibility as counselors, psychologists, social workers, and human service providers to learn about how to develop, implement, and evaluate prevention programs. Doing so will be of great service to the health and welfare of citizens.

CHAPTER 2

Basic Tenets
of Prevention

Chapter Overview

- Some Important Historical Influences
- Learning Exercise 2.1. The Broad Street Pump and Prevention
- Basic Tenets of Prevention
- Learning Exercise 2.2. Presentation: The Basic Tenets of Prevention
- Best Practice Prevention Guidelines
- Preventive Programming: Intentional and Natural
- Learning Exercise 2.3. Your Prevention Services Interview
- Summary

Every Saturday . . . a bunch of well intentioned do-gooders line up in front of my house to give away food. And it drives me crazy. (Wessels, 2008, p. 5)

The quotation above refers to volunteers from a suburban church who hand out food every Saturday in an inner-city neighborhood to those who need it. Are prevention goals served when food is given charitably and freely to people who are homeless? The answer depends on how one views prevention. Wessels suggests the answer is "no." He admits that participating in this way is a noble act that provides a portion of food for those needing it while helping those handing out the food to feel that they are helping. Unwittingly, however, handouts also may perpetuate hunger and the cycle of poverty. What do you think about this?

> At any rate, he suggests a different approach: It is time that groups work together, from both within the neighborhood and those concerned enough to come down who really want to help. It would be better, however, if the help were actually aimed at making a lasting difference—not a feel-good couple of hours satisfying some mission requirement, which is the way it seems to me. (Wessels, 2008, p. 5)

This viewpoint, expressed in a community newspaper, is provocative. In fact, however, its main theme is quite in line with current thinking of professional experts about prevention, with priority given to people-oriented projects that are collaborative, empowering, and sustainable and to efforts aimed at system change and social justice. Let's trace some of the history of prevention as a way to understand contemporary thinking and practice.

Some Important Historical Influences

Prevention in mental health, education, and communities rests upon basic tenets. These creeds and principles have been discussed by counseling psychologists in several contemporary sources (e.g., Conyne, 2004, 2008a; Hage et al., 2007; Horne, 2008; Kenny, Horne, Orpinas, & Reese, 2009; Reese & Vera, 2007; Romano & Hage, 2000), and they can be traced to multiple origins from a range of disciplines.

The work of Gerald Caplan (1964) in preventive psychiatry and of George Albee (e.g., 1986) in preventive aspects of psychology are among the most influential historically. They challenged the status quo of a one-to-one treatment orientation by pointing out that preventing these problems from occurring in the first place would be far more efficient and effective. Caplan and Albee, in turn, adopted much of their prevention perspective from public health and epidemiology (e.g., McMahon & Pugh, 1970) and applied it to mental health practice. In those disciplines, the concepts of prevalence (the total number of cases of a disorder), incidence (the number or the rate of development of new cases), and the characteristics of population, persons, place, and time are carefully considered and measured.

With regard to the concept of incidence, for example, Albee pointed out that only prevention can reduce the number of *new* cases of a disorder, such as depression, or of a problem, such as school dropouts. By contrast, although treatment is a valuable service, it is geared to address disorders that already have occurred. (In practice, as I pointed out in the Acknowledgment section, mental health treatment and prevention exist along the same helping continuum.) In addition to adjusting the main focus of help-giving from reparation of problems to their prevention, the public health contribution also expanded possible intervention targets from the individual through the population as well as intervention settings from the clinic office to the community.

The correction of social injustices also formed a central core of Albee's contribution to prevention. In his view, inequitable access to power and the effects of grinding social and economic conditions, such as poverty and the absence of health insurance, contributed powerfully to the development of psychological and emotional problems. To be preventive, therefore, meant to correct social injustices.

Contributions from the field of social work (Reamer, 1995) and community psychology (e.g., Price, 1974) added concepts of Person × Environment interaction, ecology, and systemic change to prevention, leveraging it to embrace the ecological systems within which people lived their lives. Cowen's (2000) work on health promotion within community psychology emphasized the importance of broadening the perspective of prevention from being restricted to the prevention of problems and dysfunctions to one that also included health promotion and the strengthening of healthy pathways. Thus, wellness and health promotion became both goals of and routes to prevention.

Emerging forces shaping prevention come from the areas of multicultural counseling (diversity emphasis), feminist theory (collaborative emphasis), positive psychology (strengths emphasis), and social justice (empowerment emphasis). These forces are described in several sources, including Kenny et al. (2009) and Prilleltensky and Nelson (2002). All of these historical and current influences converge dynamically, contributing to forming the basic tenets of prevention.

Basic tenets are core beliefs and assumptions that serve to guide and shape a practice. Understanding these basic tenets is important for many reasons. For our purposes, though, the chief one is this: In order to develop, conduct, and evaluate prevention programs, it is first necessary to understand what prevention is.

To introduce these basic tenets of prevention, I begin with two related classic stories that illustrate a cornerstone of public health epidemiology, intervening in the causes of disease to lower its incidence. Based on the work of John Snow in London during the cholera epidemics of 1849 and 1854, these accounts further emphasize the importance of environmental change as a preventive intervention.

Intervening in the Causes of Disease

In the 1849 instance, Snow studied cholera rates occurring in people who consumed water from two supply companies located at different locations along the Thames River. Taking ingenious advantage of naturally occurring circumstances, Snow was able to document that people consuming water from lines of the Southwark and Vauxhall Company suffered higher rates of cholera than those getting their water from the Lambeth Company. Documenting this pattern pointed to prevention possibilities not known previously.

In an equally famous follow-up case, Snow investigated an 1854 cholera outbreak in the Golden Square area of London. Data led him to center attention on the water pump at Broad Street, from which the general public drew water and around which the number of cholera cases was strikingly higher than in other areas. After examining and discarding other plausible explanations, it was determined that the Broad Street pump yielded tainted water leading to cholera. Removing the handle from the Broad Street pump made it impossible to draw water from the polluted source. This simple environmental change, following careful epidemiological assessment, lowered the incidence of cholera in London. (For more detailed description of Snow's preventive creativity, see McMahon & Pugh, 1970.)

The preventive intervention in the cause–disease link illustrated in Snow's early prevention work also can be used to promote health. The cartoon below simply illustrates the life-supporting value of clean drinking water that can pour forth from a clean water source.

Take a turn now at applying the Broad Street pump episode to prevention in mental health and education.

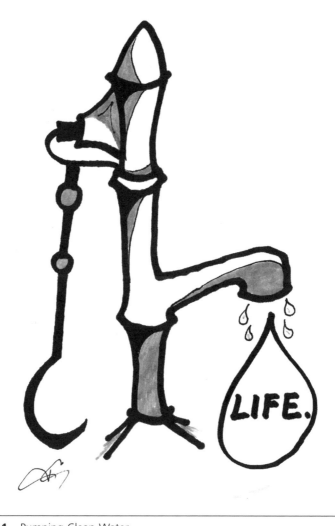

Figure 2.1 Pumping Clean Water
Source: © John Conyne.

LEARNING EXERCISE 2.1

The Broad Street Pump and Prevention

Consider John Snow's Broad Street pump experiment. Think about it in relation to prevention in mental health and education. Jot down three examples of how that experiment relates to mental health or to education:

Example 1:

_____

_____

_____

Example 2:

_____

_____

_____

Example 3:

_____

_____

_____

Test out your ideas by talking with another person.

Basic Tenets of Prevention

I suspect that some of you already have a clear grasp of prevention. For you this chapter can serve as a refresher, or you may want to skim it and move ahead. However, if research is correct that approximately 70% of counseling psychology and counselor education programs do not teach prevention (Matthews, 2003, 2004), then many of you should find this chapter helpful in providing a useful introduction to important prevention concepts.

I was asked to participate in a program at the 2008 American Psychological Association convention held in Boston (Horne, 2008) that was concerned with identifying what we know and do not know about prevention. This program was intended to serve as a kind of prevention status report. Much of the contents of this chapter are adapted from my presentation in that program (Conyne, 2008a).

Affecting Incidence

Let us start with incidence, an essential prevention concept. *Incidence* is a public health term (McMahon & Pugh, 1970) that refers to halting the emergence of *new* cases (or the rate of development of new cases) of any targeted disorder or problem. Incidence reduction occurs, for instance, when the number of new cases of dropouts in a school decreases. Incidence reduction is the "gold standard" of prevention. If new cases of a disorder can be stopped or slowed, then the need for more expensive reparative activity also is diminished and—more importantly—the breadth and depth of human suffering is lowered.

Prevention can stop problems from occurring. At its most elemental form, prevention can be thought of as a stop sign. Preventing, or stopping, the traffic of a problem, such as school bullying, is the purest kind of prevention. In this view, when something is prevented, it is stopped, or at least the rate of emergence of new cases of this problem is retarded.

Affecting Prevalence

Prevalence also is a public health term. It refers to the total number of cases of a dysfunction, disorder, or problem. This amount results from the number of new cases of the disorder and the number of already existing cases of that same disorder. Prevalence is the product of incidence and duration, expressed as: Prevalence = Incidence × Duration, or $P = I \times D$. It includes concepts of incidence (the number of new cases) and of duration and severity (the condition of continuing cases). Thinking about these three elements helps to distinguish the emphases of prevention from those of remediation or treatment, as follows:

- Prevention is intended to lower incidence of new cases.
- Treatment is intended to lower duration and severity of already existing cases.
- Prevalence can be reduced by lowering incidence, duration, and/or incidence and duration of current cases.

The next three applications of prevention (delaying onset, reducing duration, and reducing severity) affect problems once they have emerged. If effective, they can serve to lower the prevalence of the problem, that is, the overall numbers of it at any time.

Prevention can delay the onset of a disorder or problem. Think of this aspect of prevention as a Yield sign. An anticipated problem is held back so that its possible occurrence arrives later. If a problem can be delayed, then opportunity is provided to strengthen resistance to it through approaches such as skill training or environmental change.

Prevention can reduce the duration of a disorder or problem. This is what has been termed *secondary prevention.* That is, the problem already is being experienced. Let's say that a manager was suddenly let go from her job, and now, 3 weeks later, she is beginning to experience a variety of negative emotional consequences. If psychological assistance, such as the JOBS Project for the Unemployed (Vinokur, Schul, Vuori, & Price, 2000), can be provided early in this process, then the continuation of these emotional consequences may be reduced.

Prevention can reduce the severity of a disorder or problem. This aspect of prevention has been termed *tertiary prevention.* Emotional and psychological pain can be intense and debilitating. Consider veterans returning from Operation Iraqi Freedom many of whom have been subjected to severe stress and violence. Once home, around 30% of them experience post-traumatic stress disorder. Prevention services, such as linking support services, can assist in moderating problem intensity.

Prevention can strengthen existing assets to promote health and well-being. Prevention programs can be aimed at identifying and enhancing existing strengths as well as developing additional strengths, including knowledge, attitudes, and skills. Reflecting this view, DeAngelis (1994) acknowledged Elias, who asserted that the absence of problems or illness is not the same as health. More recently, Keyes (2007) expounded on this perspective in his concept of "flourishing," a state of complete mental health characterized by an absence of mental illness plus positive emotions and positive psychological and social functioning.

Cowen (2000) maintained that early-wellness prevention programs can provide the best "inoculation," serving to protect against a range of future adverse conditions from which all people, not only those at risk, can benefit. He identified five wellness-enhancement strategies: (a) promote wholesome caregiver–child attachment relationships, (b) help children develop stage-appropriate competencies, (c) create environments that are wellness enhancing, (d) bolster the capacity of people to ward off stressors and manage stress, and (e) help people to become empowered.

Prevention can support organizational, institutional, community, and governmental policies and practices that enhance health and well-being. People live in contexts, surrounded by environmental forces that are physical, social, and economic that emerge locally and internationally. Some have noted that there are sick and healthy environments just as there are sick and healthy people. One of the prevention strategies for addressing negative environmental conditions is advocacy (Lewis, Arnold, House, & Toporek, 2002). One form of advocacy targets noxious public policies or environmental conditions as the focus for change that, if successful, can potentially benefit the lives of those affected.

Holding a "Prevention Perspective" Is Essential

In the opinion of many experts, holding a "prevention perspective" overshadows all else in enabling a practitioner to become involved with prevention. A prevention perspective is qualitatively distinct from the remedial viewpoint that dominates training, practice, and the perceptions of legislators, funding bodies, and the general public.

Before-the-Fact Orientation. A before-the-fact orientation represents the lens of prevention. By viewing the world through this lens, a practitioner actually sees psychological and emotional events and experiences differently than usual. This is analogous to, let's say, a high-definition digital signal compared to the analog one, or color television compared to black and white. Clarity and hue aren't at issue as much as being able to see entirely different reasons, sequences, and relationships for the emergence of problems and how to address them. Think of putting on "before-the-fact lenses" much as you might put on special glasses at a 3-D movie. Now a whole new way of viewing becomes possible. With regard to psychological and emotional dysfunction, for example, putting on a set of before-the-fact lenses affects all that you view because it focuses the following vision: being able to see problems as preventable, before they take effect, or at least very early in their progression.

Incidence Reduction. This "gold standard" of prevention, referred to above, represents the ultimate goal for any project. It is part and parcel of the before-the-fact orientation. We always desire to stop the emergence of new cases of a problem in its tracks. However, caution is needed here and perhaps some nuance, too, due to the complexity of psychological and emotional problems. In most disorders, such as depression, cause-and-effect relationships are typically not singular and linear. That is, there is no uniform straight line that can be drawn. Rather, combinations of personal and environmental strengths and deficits interact over time. (I realize what you've just read is quite a mouthful. Hold on, we will be breaking these concepts down more simply as we move ahead.) Resulting interactions may lead to depression (or some other disorder) in one person, to substance abuse in another, or to no discernable dysfunction in yet a third person.

At any rate, incidence reduction can be approached through programs that coordinate efforts to lower deficits while increasing strengths (Albee, 1985; Bloom, 1996). Albee's incidence reduction formula involves decreasing deficits in the numerator while increasing strengths in the denominator. It is depicted as follows:

$$\text{Reducing Incidence} = \frac{\text{Decrease } \textbf{Deficits} \text{ (Organic Factors} + \text{Stress} + \text{Exploitation)}}{\text{Increase } \textbf{Strengths} \text{ (Self-Esteem} + \text{Coping Skills} + \text{Support Groups)}}$$

This formula will be described in detail later. With some adaptation, it will be relied upon as a primary guide for developing and evaluating prevention programs.

Healthy Targets. It must be clear by now that prevention is not prevention if programs are intended for people who are coping with diagnosable dysfunctions or who are entrenched in other forms of adjustment problems. Having said that, an argument can be made that prevention also involves helping those who are presently diagnosed with one condition from developing other conditions, for instance, preventing persons with anorexia from also becoming depressed. Although that approach is viable in practice, it is not what is generally considered to be prevention. Health promotion prevention programs are universal in scope, emphasizing enhancement of healthy functioning in a population of people, whether or not they may be at risk for any particular dysfunction.

An example is the Voices Against Violence prevention program at the University of Texas at Austin. Program goals include raising awareness about relationship violence and sexual assault, counseling survivors, and changing the campus culture (Meyers, 2008). This campus-wide program is aimed at all freshmen, as well as others on campus, and a variety of components include training, outreach, and advocacy. A powerful aspect is the peer theater group that seeks to stimulate audience and performer dialogue about pertinent social issues through its performances. Such prevention programs are intended for all in the community, assuming that everyone is at some risk, even if it is a relatively small increment (J. McWhirter, McWhirter, McWhirter, & McWhirter, 1995).

Ecological/Systems Analysis. Prevention programs typically take place in natural settings rather than in clinic offices—in schools, communities, families, at work, and in other commonplace locations. By definition, these are not experimental laboratories where variables can be more readily manipulated and controlled. In fact, the opposite situation applies. Conditions and variables in settings where prevention occurs tend to be dynamic and interactive, and come in multiple forms and levels.

Consider developing and conducting an academic support program in an inner-city school, for instance. An often unpredictable and changing environment might constitute the context, subject to shifting resources, uncertain community and parent involvement, variable attendance patterns, and scheduling conflicts (to identify a few possible challenges). Prevention programs, then, need to be designed following broad and ongoing assessment of personal and situational variables and how they interact over time. An ecological-systemic analysis (Chronister, McWhirter, & Kerewsky, 2004; Conyne & Clack, 1981; Conyne & Cook, 2004) is well suited to these conditions.

Multiplicity: Elements, Methods, and Levels. Implicit within an ecological-systemic analysis is the concept of multiplicity. Prevention is accomplished by addressing and attempting to influence multiple elements, using multiple methods, and applied through multiple levels (Dryfoos, 1997; Nation et al., 2003). Recall the incidence reduction formula of Albee, presented earlier. Note that in its numerator and denominator there are a number of elements. Effective prevention programs need to be based on an assessment of these elements, drawn from personal and environmental domains, with those that may represent strengths as well as deficits. Then, prevention programs usually include a number of methods to affect these elements. Among other possibilities, these might involve consultation, training, psychoeducation, group work, and advocacy. Depending on the project, these methods may be applied at any of several levels: individual, group, family, organization, community, governmental, and so on. The interplay of these multiple factors will be addressed when we focus later on prevention program development and evaluation.

Collaboration. The creation and delivery of prevention programs tilts horizontally, not vertically. By this I mean that a vertical style, which can be described as being top down, autocratically driven, and one way, is avoided in favor of a horizontal direction—lateral, democratic, and based on co-expert/co-learner cooperation (Elden & Levin, 1991). As Rappaport cogently observed decades ago, in prevention it is desirable to *work with* people, not to *do to* them (Rappaport, 1981). Working with people by sharing and applying mutual sets of expertise—collaborating—takes advantage of a broader range of resources while flattening out power issues. This type of equalitarian participation is not always easy to accomplish. However, it can yield satisfaction and outcomes benefiting both local practice and the community of science.

Social Justice

In addition to applying the concept of incidence reduction to mental health, another seminal contribution of George Albee to prevention centered on programs that tackled social injustice. He held that mental health disorders were multicausal, with inequities existing within society contributing substantially. Albee suggested that the redistribution of social power was an important means for advancing social justice, with organic factors playing a lesser role. The following view of Albee is instructive:

> We are concerned with problems in living, problems often created by blows of fate, by the damaging forces of a racist, sexist, ageist society where preparation for competent adaptation is minimal. (Albee, 1980, cited in Albee & Gullotta, 1997, p. 25)

Achieving increased levels of social justice, he reasoned, would exert preventive effects, promoting healthier functioning. This social justice approach to prevention is held as a cornerstone tenet among many theorists today (Vera & Spreight, 2003). For example, the forthcoming volume *Realizing Social Justice* (Kenny et al., 2009) centers on how preventive interventions can be used. In this perspective, prevention is a key strategy for challenging social structures and policies that serve to restrict access to power and to resources according to ethnicity, race, gender, or religion (Davidson, Waldo, & Adams, 2006; Lee, 2007; Toporek, Gerstein, Fouad, Roysircar, & Israel, 2006).

However, social justice is not without its critics. Hunsaker (2008), for example, challenges what he views as a strident, liberal political agenda of social justice and rejects its value for counseling. In my opinion, incorporating a social justice approach always has been an essential part of prevention, and it does not mean that strategies aimed at increasing personal competency and responsibility are ignored or undervalued. Both approaches are valuable and important.

Cultural Relevance

Incorporating cultural relevance within prevention programs tends to strengthen those efforts (Mercy, Krug, Dahlberg, & Zwi, 2003). Such programs are designed and conducted to be consistent with the "values, beliefs, and desired outcomes of a particular community" (Reese & Vera, 2007).

The most effective culturally relevant prevention programs involve program participants in the major phases of the program: its design, implementation, and evaluation (Reiss & Price, 1996). In other instances, when participants are involved in substantively adapting an existing and effective prevention program, "deep structure modifications" (Resnicow, Solar, Braithwaite, Ahluwalia, & Butler, 2000) can result, where the changed program components may not resemble the original program in all respects. This alteration has two effects: (a) It allows the adapted program to be reflective of local circumstances and may serve to increase participant involvement and adherence, and (b) it leads to research and evaluation challenges because the adapted program is not the same one as the tested model.

These two effects combine to form a creative tension between local relevance and science that is the subject of both excitement and concern. Griffin and Miller (2007), for instance, after reviewing a number of culturally relevant prevention programs (Reese & Vera, 2007; Vera et al., 2007), suggest that an operational definition of cultural relevance be developed, accompanied by the structural components of culturally relevant prevention programs that are minimally required to produce effective and replicable intervention protocols. Griffin and Miller (2007, p. 853) cautioned that such an evidence-based, culturally relevant quest should not depress the incorporation of innovation and new ideas into the program design process. Seeking the "perfect" (evidence-based), they said, should not be the enemy of the "good" (evolving programs being tested).

Empowerment

Prevention programs are intended to empower people and systems (Conyne, 2004). When people are empowered, they are able to access opportunities and resources. They are self-efficacious, enjoy more control over their personal lot in life, and can positively influence life situations they face. Ellen McWhirter (1994) conceptualized an empowerment approach to counseling, where people, groups, or organizations that are powerless or are marginalized are helped to gain strength and competency. She maintains that people become more empowered when they realize how power dynamics affect their lives, how they can gain greater control over their lives without infringing on others, and how they can help empower others in the community.

LEARNING EXERCISE 2.2

Presentation: The Basic Tenets of Prevention

You've just been introduced to some basic tenets of prevention.

Assume you have been asked to give a 15-minute presentation to the Annual Conference on Prevention on the topic "The Basic Tenets of Prevention." Prepare an outline of your remarks below. Then, actually give the presentation to a friend or fellow student.

Outline your remarks:

_____

_____

_____

Best Practice Prevention Guidelines

Best practice guidelines in prevention have been developed to influence the preventive functioning of psychologists in research, practice, training, and social advocacy (Hage et al., 2007). They also can serve to summarize the basic tenets discussed throughout this chapter. The guidelines encourage psychologists (and, by implication, other helping professionals) who are interested in prevention to

1. Use proactive interventions to prevent distress and human suffering.

2. Select interventions that are based on theory and supported by evidence.

3. Apply culturally relevant practices that involve relevant participants in all planning and programming phases.

4. Develop interventions that include individual and contextual/systemic factors contributing to well-being and to psychological dysfunction.

5. Implement interventions that are intended to reduce risks and promote strengths across the life span.

6. View practice within ongoing developments in prevention science.

7. Establish competence in research methods appropriate for prevention research.

8. Conduct research that is in accord with environmental contexts.

9. Be mindful of ethical issues connected with prevention research.

10. Consider social justice implications of prevention research.

11. Develop knowledge of concepts and research in prevention and of skills in prevention practice and scholarship.

12. Foster awareness, knowledge, and skills of prevention required in psychological education and training.

13. Design, promote, and support systemic initiatives lowering the incidence of psychological and physical dysfunction.

14. Design, promote, and support institutional change strategies enhancing the health and well-being of individuals, families, and communities.

15. Engage in advocacy activities within governmental, legislative, and political arenas to strengthen the health and well-being of the wider population being served.

Prevention Programming: Intentional and Natural

Nike's famous injunction—"Just Do It"—while possessing motivational properties, certainly oversimplifies life. Premier athletes hone their gifted bodies through intensely focused and persistent trial and training occurring over years in order to compete. Getting out the door for a jog for many people is itself complicated, not defined by spontaneous activity. Leaving the athletic metaphor and turning for a moment to eating, I am stunned every Thanksgiving when my wife produces a feast fit for royalty, and I know from washing the dishes that this was no simple act.

So it is with any mental health or educational approach. Putting theory into practice requires knowledge, skill, and sensitivity. Because mental health prevention is multifaceted, its execution typically requires the intentional coordination of many factors.

Yet as we have seen from the first chapter, the prevention of pernicious factors and conditions can occur naturally—as through applying the Ruby and Oren Principle that underscores the value of social connections—or it can spring as a kind of side effect from programs that have been designed to affect entirely other factors.

Examples of such programs can be found in a variety of areas, including sports and the arts. In our own case in the University of Cincinnati Counseling Program, we collaborated in a preventive effort with the Inner City Youth Opportunities collaborative (ICYO, http://www.icyo.us/ICYO.pdf), a developmental asset-building community program that uses tennis as a vehicle to intentionally enhance self-esteem, encourage goal setting, develop anger-management skills, and promote academic achievement.

In the arts, consider "El Sistema," or "The System" in English (O'Keefe, 2007; Radcliffe, 2008). It is a classical music training program for children in Venezuela that has produced world-class artists and is said to have contributed to improved citizenship and to the lowering of poverty, crime, and untimely gang deaths. Over its 30 years of existence as a community classical music training program, El Sistema has taught 250,000 Venezuelan children coming from the most remote rural country villages and the poorest barrios of Caracas. Its founder and director, Joseph Antonio Abrieu, envisioned that musical training could overcome the "spiritual poverty" that can accompany economic and social inequities, so that students gain not only musical skills (with several being placed in major orchestras around the world) but skills in living that can help them to overcome their disadvantaged backgrounds. As such, El Sistema functions as both an artistic and a social change project that is being emulated in countries throughout the world.

Another example of a naturally based program is Therapeutic Lifestyle Change (TLC), which is intended to treat depression (Ilardi et al., 2007; Ilardi & Karwoski, 2005, cited in Snyder & Lopez, 2007, pp. 365–366; www.psych.ku.edu/tlc). Implemented prior to the onset of depression, it also would seem that applying the program's components could provide a preventive effect. The TLC program is based on the premise that our modern, high-tech lifestyles have served to move us too far away from the natural lives of our ancestors, which were based on ongoing and active connections with the environment and with others.

The TLC program, which is delivered through a group format, has been found to be as effective as medication in treating depression. Its six lifestyle components are: (a) exercising aerobically at least three times per week, 30 minutes each time; (b) obtaining light exposure of at least 30 minutes per day; (c) ingesting omega-3 fatty acids or supplements; (d) engaging in social support, spending as much time with others as possible; (e) using anti-rumination strategies, such as running or challenging negative thoughts, that are aimed at combating persistent worrying; and (f) sleeping at least 8 hours per night.

Prevention programs, then, need to be carefully planned and take advantage of natural circumstance and resources. These are among the basic tenets of prevention.

But how can you distinguish a prevention program from other mental health approaches? Consider the following learning exercise.

LEARNING EXERCISE 2.3

Your Prevention Services Interview

Yes, prevention programming in mental health and education lags behind treatment approaches. But, certainly, prevention is occurring in our schools and mental health centers, in the workplace, and in communities—to mention a few important settings. I'd like you to explore a sampling of your local environment to discover the status of preventive services. Here's how:

Over the next month, make a contact with one local school and one mental health agency. Arrange for a 30-minute appointment with a professional staff person. Then conduct an interview and note what you find. You might follow the steps below:

A. *Interview*

- Introduce yourself.
- Describe your purpose: You are reading a book on prevention, and you are wanting to learn about their services and programs.
- Thank them for the interview.
- Make summary notes of your interview.

B. *Analysis*

- Apply prevention definitions and criteria to analyze programs and services offered.
- What, if any, are preventive in intent?
- Why?

Once a prevention program or service is being delivered, how can you determine if the program is a good one? Are there basic criteria that exist to help? Now that we have focused on the basic tenets upon which prevention rests, we can move naturally to this next question of criteria for determining prevention. These topics will be considered in the next chapter.

Summary

Prevention exceeds folklore and bromides, of course. This chapter built on the notions about everyday prevention discussed in Chapter 1. It traced some of prevention's important historical evolution and then described a number of basic tenets upon which it rests. These tenets are: (a) definition of prevention, including incidence, prevalence, and other elements; (b) prevention perspective, embracing before-the-fact time frame, incidence reduction mind-set, ecological-systemic assessment, multiplicity of programs, and collaboration; (c) social justice value; (d) the importance of cultural relevance; and (e) empowerment as a goal.

Best practice guidelines for prevention practice, research, training, and social advocacy were discussed because of their capacity to guide effective and ethical prevention work. Prevention programs typically require focused, intentional, and coordinated program development procedures following best practices. However, it also was noted in this chapter that prevention can and does occur by amplifying natural processes, such as in the TLC program, and as a powerful side effect of programs that target other main goals, such as in El Sistema.

CHAPTER 3

Criteria for Determining a Prevention Program

In this chapter we will focus on criteria for determining a prevention program. Criteria assist in knowing what prevention is and what it is not. These criteria, then, can help guide both program development and program evaluation. When I work with students or trainees in prevention, we spend a lot of time becoming familiar with criteria and then applying them against prevention programs that have been evaluated as "excellent." I ask them: "What makes these programs excellent?" Students work in small groups to apply these criteria in seeking to answer the question. When we begin to consider developing and evaluating prevention programs, these criteria also serve to ground that effort.

The criteria that follow are informed by the meta-analyses cited in the previous chapter, as well as from other sources. The first eight intervention criteria presented are adapted from the "review of reviews" by Nation et al. (2003). This is a good place to begin.

Broad Criteria for Determining Prevention Programs

Comprehensiveness

Effective prevention programs are comprehensive in scope. They tend to be longer term and sometimes longitudinal, address protective and risk factors, and include person-centered and system-centered components. Each of these areas is discussed below.

Longer Term. "Single-shot" prevention presentations—that is, those that are presented briefly and for one time, such as a 1-hour lecture on preventing stress or a 2-hour workshop on that topic—typically are unable to produce sustainable preventive effects. Longer-term programs are more likely to effect growth and change, but length alone is not sufficient. For instance, prevention programs conducted over a longer time period but that are limited to one domain, such as a knowledge or skill area, possess limited potency.

Protective and Risk Factors. By contrast, effective prevention programs tend to be both longer term and comprehensive, echoing the basic tenet of multiplicity discussed earlier. These programs typically include several planned interventions aimed to accomplish interlacing goals revolving around increasing protective factors (strengths) while decreasing risk factors (deficits). For example, in a substance abuse prevention program aimed at teenagers, protective factor interventions might include presentation of cognitive information to increase awareness and knowledge, psychoeducation skill development segments to develop resistance skills, and pairing participants with mentors to provide ongoing support. Risk reduction factors in the same program might target reduction of stressors in teens' lives, advocating for increased resources to address teenage substance abuse, and educational campaigns aimed at parents to instruct them in how to eliminate home access by teenagers to unprescribed and over-the-counter medicines.

Person Centered and System Centered. In addition to a multimodal approach, successful prevention programs are focused broadly to include members of the targeted population (person centered) but also settings, situations, and environments that are relevant and influential (system centered). Person-centered aspects of a substance abuse prevention program might target parents, school personnel, and peers, while system-centered components might address aspects of environments, such as their physical properties, policies, and procedures. As has been pointed out (e.g., Conyne, 2004; Hawkins & Catalano, 1992), a range of factors needs to be addressed across domains or settings that have main impact on the program participants.

Direct Experiencing Methods

Effective prevention interventions tend to be interactive, involving participants in direct, hands-on experience (Tobler et al., 2000; Tobler & Stratton, 1997). After reviewing three meta-analyses for school-based adolescent drug prevention programs, Tobler (2000) found that noninteractive prevention programs produced a 4% reduction in prevalence rates while interactive programs yielded a 21% reduction. She concluded that small, interactive programs were the more successful. Such findings favoring direct experience have been found in a broad range of areas, cautioning against prevention programs that emphasize one-way transmission or group discussion of knowledge and information rather than highlighting skill development and other forms of direct participation and experience.

Sufficient Dosage

Successful prevention programs provide enough potency to produce intended effects. Termed *sufficient dosage*, or the intensity of the intervention, this concept in prevention is not unlike what we might ordinarily think of when treating a cold, where the dosage size of cough syrup is measured. I think of sufficient dosage as applying the so-called "Goldilocks Rule," adapted from the fairy tale *Goldilocks and the Three Bears*. Those of you with long memories may remember how Goldilocks entered a house in the forest, looking to find the porridge, chair, and bed that were "just right." Not too hot or cold (porridge), not too big or too little (chair), and not too hard or soft (bed). In each case she sorted through options that were too this or too that, until finding the ones that were—again—"just right."

Prevention programs that are just right in dosage typically are measured by such considerations as the number, frequency, and length of each session, the overall brevity or length of the program, and the amount, kind, and expense of resources employed. Because some research has indicated that the durability of prevention effects may wither over time (e.g., Zigler, Taussig, & Black, 1992), "booster sessions" can be used in an attempt to sustain them. These follow-up sessions, analogous to vaccination boosters, renew attention to knowledge and skills that were conveyed initially in the program. The booster session concept in prevention programs is borrowed from medical practice, where a booster shot in the arm is readministered to continue the potency of an originally dispensed vaccine. Botvin's work in substance abuse prevention makes excellent use of such booster sessions (e.g., Botvin, Baker, Dusenbury, Botvin, & Diaz, 1995).

Theory Driven

Effective prevention programs typically arise from theoretical guidance rather than experience or common sense, although the latter two factors sometimes too strongly characterize prevention efforts. The "science of prevention" (Coie et al., 1993) is a logical and sequential framework that illustrates one form of a theory-driven approach. It is etiology (cause) based. Preventive interventions are inserted between the chain of events assessed as linking risk and prospective disorder. This causal-link model, however, works better with certain public health initiatives than with mental health. Smallpox eradication offers magnificent testimony to public health success. On the other hand, the prevention of malaria, for instance, remains a daunting and significant challenge in certain areas of the Americas, Asia, and Africa, despite a causal link: Find and treat the source (e.g., swamps) that gives rise to agents (female mosquitoes) that transmit the protozoan parasite to the host (humans) who then contracts the disease. Theoretically, at least, swamps can be drained, mosquitoes can be controlled or eliminated, and people can take precautions such as using mosquito nets when living in or visiting settings for which malarial infection is an identified risk. The reality being confronted in underdeveloped environments where malaria (and tuberculosis and AIDS) run wildly amok is highly resistive to such efforts due to a foreboding set of reasons that lay outside this discussion.

Etiology and effect are often unclear when mental health prevention is concerned, as there usually are numerous pathways through which risk and disorder may be associated. Moreover, a set of certain circumstances (e.g., absent father, child abuse) can lead to a wide range of dysfunction (e.g., school failure, hostility, substance abuse) rather than one that might be anticipated, or to none at all (Conyne, 2004).

Another set of theories, termed *intervention theories* (Nation et al., 2003), address the most effective ways to change or reduce these causal links. Positive Youth Development, multicultural psychology, social learning, developmental psychology, positive psychology, and social justice represent some of the bodies of knowledge that are important in mental health prevention (Kenny & Romano, 2009). Theoretical models that address individual-level factors have found utility in guiding prevention programs, such as the health belief model, theory of reasoned action, and attribution theory. Recently, ecological and developmental contextual theory have assumed importance and relevance in conceptualizing and delivering prevention programs (Reese, Wingfield, & Blumenthal, 2009; Walsh, DePaul, & Park-Taylor, in press). These theories emphasize how multiple personal and contextual factors influence development across the life span.

Two theories addressing readiness for change that have been used largely in psychotherapy and addictions treatment but that hold potential for prevention are the transtheoretical stages of change approach (Prochaska & DiClemente, 2005), which I referred to earlier, and motivational interviewing (Rollnick & Miller, 1995). In the first approach, intervention is geared to mesh appropriately with the pertinent stage of client readiness for change. These stages include pre-contemplation ("never thought about it"), contemplation ("beginning to think about it"), preparation ("planning to act"), action ("taking steps"), maintenance ("continuing commitment"), and—too often—relapse ("backsliding"). Motivational interviewing also places high importance on a client's readiness and ambivalence about change, using client-centered, relationship-oriented approaches in an effort to help clients choose if and how to move ahead with change.

Provide Opportunities for Positive Relationships

Prevention programs that are successful, as has been pointed out, tend to be interactive and involve direct experience. Implied is that direct interaction will spawn new positive relationships and strengthen any existing ones. Impactful programs accentuate human capital, intensifying connections among people and empowering them to fuller functioning (Conyne, 2004). In the case of prevention programs for children, reviews also have pointed to the value of providing opportunities for kids to develop improved relationships with parents and peers, and with significant others in relevant systems—such as teachers in school. Carefully selected mentors can provide this kind of connection (Grossman & Tierney, 1998).

Appropriately Timed

Teachers-in-training all learn about the concept of the "teachable moment." Students are more open to learning and change at certain developmental points in their lives or when certain conditions occur than at other times. For instance, two middle school students become embroiled in a yelling match on the school playground. Observing the event, the supervising teacher intervenes, seeking to convert the yelling match into a teachable moment by stopping the action and introducing the two students to a helpful coping skills strategy developed by Horne (2005), whose suggested steps form the acronym SCIDDLE (Stop, Calm down, Identify the issue, Decide what to do, Do it, Look around to see what happens, and Evaluate how it works). At this point of real-world conflict, learning and applying the model has the advantage of being timed appropriately. Conversely, teaching the coping skills strategy abstractly in class or in a training session, while still of benefit, cannot take advantage of the naturally occurring event.

Another popular phrase, "It's all in the timing," applies to many situations. It can refer to profitable stock trading, the syncopation of jazz, the stroke of a successful hitter in baseball, and to the immediacy of effective feedback—as well as to prevention programs. Such programs need to be developmentally timed and appropriate in order to work. Kids and adults are developmentally ready for qualitatively different kinds of knowledge and skills. Expecting 5-year-old children to function in open-ended group sessions is unrealistic developmentally, but this may be appropriate for adults.

Because a preventive program is intended to be delivered "before the fact" (or as early as possible in problem development), it is advisable to time its delivery prior to disorder or problem onset. In an obvious case, but to make the point, a program to prevent students from dropping out of school needs to be made available to students who are still in school but may be at risk for this eventuality.

Culturally Relevant

Prevention programs also need to be tailored appropriately to participants' developmental and cultural characteristics. Tailoring programs to fit levels of intellectual, cognitive, and social functioning and to the cultural values of participants helps to assure program acceptance and involvement, if not success. You might consider how a prevention program based on social support could be designed to fit participants who are older rather than younger, that comprises Hispanics versus whites, or that is located in an impoverished rural setting versus a wealthy suburban one.

Ethnicity, race, and culture combine to powerfully shape contexts. How psychological problems and strengths are expressed in these different contexts should be understood and included within prevention program design and execution. Doing so requires applying a culture-centered perspective giving credence to group and individual characteristics such as age, gender, race, ethnicity, abilities, religion, sexual orientation, language, immigration status, socioeconomic status, and others (Gottfredson, Fink, Skroban, & Gottfredson, 1997). Moreover, the participation of representatively diverse stakeholders needs to be included genuinely and collaboratively throughout program design, implementation, and evaluation (Kenny et al., 2009; Kenny & Romano, 2009).

Competent Staff

Prevention programs that are researched and designed effectively, of course, are dependent on equally effective implementation. Without well-trained staff to implement the program, the probability for success is reduced. These staff need not be professionally trained or licensed, however. In fact, staff who represent the program participants along at least some obvious dimensions (e.g., ethnicity, race, age, gender, cultural ties) bring with them a kind of local expertise that can make an especially powerful contribution. A program I was involved with at the Illinois State University Student Counseling Service used college student paraprofessional peer students as helpers, psychoeducation workshop presenters, and campus environmental assessors. Closely trained and supervised, this student-to-student delivery format was experienced as authentic and was well received by other students.

As mentioned, competent staff must be trained but, also, they need to be supported and supervised (Lewis, Battistich, & Schaps, 1990, cited in Nation et al., 2003). Support is often particularly important. I have supervised numerous projects in schools, universities, and neighborhoods where most necessary conditions for effective application were in place except for maintaining staff continuity. A lack of resources sometimes accounts for turnover, but often, failure to sustain an accessible and meaningful system of support seemed more potent.

Readiness of the Setting

This concept applies timing to the setting in which the program will be delivered. Because prevention programs are usually delivered in situ, it is necessary to consider setting readiness. Referred to usually as "community readiness," use of the term *setting* allows for a broader understanding, inclusive of communities, schools, work places, and other host environments. The essential concept, however, is that any setting must be ready in order for a setting-based prevention program to work.

Terroir is a French term containing many shades of meaning that vintners (winemakers) apply to grape-growing conditions. I learned about this term during a tour of some California wineries. It seems that producing quality wines requires a positive terroir, where environmental conditions such as soil composition, moisture, sun, time, and temperature (and, no doubt, more) all interact harmoniously to nurture grape health and growth. Particular terroirs give rise to certain wine types and to overall wine quality. Environmental threats to terroir (e.g., harsh temperatures or short rainfall amounts) result in conditions that are unready to stimulate and support wine yield, resulting in lower productivity and an inferior wine.

In some respects, good prevention programs are like a good, complex wine. (You may never have thought of them that way!) Wine depends on grapes to take root, prosper, and be processed. The conditions need to be supportive and ready. So, too, with prevention programs. Several factors help to determine setting readiness for prevention: (a) Sufficient setting capacity is available; (b) setting members recognize that a problem or need exists; (c) members realize that any current programs or efforts are not enough; (d) an appropriate climate for implementation exists; and (e) a key champion for program installation is identified (Stith et al., 2006). With regard to problem and need recognition (point b, above), for instance, one set of researchers (Edwards, Jumper-Thurman, Plested, Oetting, & Swanson, 2000; Oetting et al., 1995) identified nine stages, ranging from no awareness at all of a problem or need for prevention (Stage 1); through preparation (Stage 5), where planning and operational details have been accomplished and a trial prevention program has begun; to professionalization (Stage 9), where prevention efforts are fully defined and supported, staff training is in place, and setting members participate actively.

The Agency for Healthcare Research and Quality (AHRQ, 2008a) of the U.S. Department of Health and Human Services maintains a program, *Put Prevention Into Practice* (PPIP). A key PPIP component is concerned with staff and organizational readiness for prevention. A number of assessment products available through PPIP are useful, but the two most germane for this discussion of readiness are: (a) *Readiness Survey,* to ascertain staff attitudes, and (b) *Worksheet for Assessing Organizational Climate,* to describe the setting's suitability for prevention.

To give you a sense of how readiness is assessed in each instrument, excerpts are presented next. Staff respond to each of the 16 Readiness Survey statements by using a 7-point scale (1 = Very much; 7 = Not at all). The first 3 Readiness Survey statements are:

1. Prevention is an important aspect of the care we provide in this practice.

2. We think prevention should be more strongly emphasized in our practice.

3. Someone in our practice has the vision, leadership, and authority to make prevention happen here.

The Worksheet for Assessing Organizational Climate asks setting members to describe their values, attitudes, and beliefs about prevention, as well as those of their patients, and whether staff perceive a need for change and are ready to institute change. Resulting qualitative information is summarized and used to determine if prevention programming may be indicated.

Build Effective Collaborative Community Partnerships

Prevention programs, as you have read, are typically conducted within external settings, not in a clinic office. By definition, community-based programs demand a community-based approach. Another way to state this is that it takes a team to do prevention. Therefore, effective collaborative community partnerships need to be established, which can then serve as guiding forces for prevention program development, implementation, and evaluation.

Steps have been identified for creating such team-based partnerships (e.g., Stith et al., 2006). These steps include attending to developing, leading, maintaining, and evaluating the partnership. For instance, if communication among partnership members is characterized by "turf wars" and disrespect, then the strength of the partnership is jeopardized, with the capacity to guide the prevention program compromised.

Participation of prevention specialists in this entire process requires careful consideration. A collaborative and co-expert model fits well with community partnerships (Elden & Levin, 1991; Jacobson & Rugeley, 2007), as I discussed in the preceding chapter. In such an approach community and professional partners cooperate laterally, with each contributing unique and complementary expertise. Dumka, Mauricio, and Gonzales (2007) illustrate this approach well in describing how a school advisory board was used in their *Puentes* prevention program with Mexican-origin families.

Deliver With Fidelity and With Fit

Fidelity in relationships is a prized virtue. One who demonstrates it is thought to be loyal, devoted, faithful, and capable of allegiance. These qualities attend to delivering a prevention program with fidelity, too. In addition, the qualities of exactness and integrity apply. A program is delivered with fidelity when it is presented in accord with how it was intended. It can be trusted. Evidence-based programs (those that are buttressed by effectiveness and clinical support) that are delivered with fidelity tend to produce more positive outcomes than do programs lacking evidence and fidelity (Dusenbury & Hansen, 2004; D. Elliott & Mihalic, 2004; Zaza, Briss, & Harris, 2005).

Yet you might wonder, what about adaptation and flexibility during program delivery, where changing conditions might be met with changing program components or styles? How about adapting a proven program to fit local cultural differences or to mesh more closely with particular participant needs or setting characteristics? For example, given the stricture of fidelity, is it legitimate to shape a proven program to anticipate ethnic features of a unique population?

Certainly, arguments exist for intentionally modifying program regimens to sensitively address local conditions, including such considerations as differential developmental risk, age level, setting resources, and multicultural dimensions (Castro, Barrera, & Martinez, 2004; Collins, Murphy, & Bierman, 2004; Stith et al., 2006). This perspective prioritizes the fit of a program over its fidelity. Culturally relevant approaches, for example, have generally been found to yield higher participant acceptance, involvement, and satisfaction than those that are generic (Reese et al., 2009), produce programs that are more relevant to participants (Nation et al., 2003), and can improve recruitment, retention, and outcome effectiveness (Kumpfer, Alvarado, Smith, & Bellamy, 2002; Reese, Vera, Simon, & Ikeda, 2000). Opposing arguments (e.g., D. Elliott & Mihalic, 2004; Pentz, 2004) suggest that program implementation deviating from proven design and implementation steps, either purposefully or spontaneously, diminishes program effectiveness and complicates the interpretation of results. Kelly (2004) considers how inadequate program replication can usurp the effect of an evidence-based intervention. Stith et al. (2006) summarize a number of strategies to increase fidelity even when engaging in adaptations of efficacious prevention programs, and Byrd and Reininger (2009) helpfully describe one approach in detail.

Drawn from several sources, strategies to increase both fidelity and fit include: (a) Identify and include the core components of the program that cannot be altered or adapted, (b) build in adaptations to fit local conditions without threatening the core components of the program, (c) seek to reach maximum adherence and dosage, (d) integrate ongoing feedback and supervision related to program implementation, (e) supply adequate staff training and supervision, (f) assess and address roadblocks that threaten implementation fidelity, and (g) design the program for feasibility so that it can be conducted and maintained in the real world, which is replete with constraints.

Groups

Prevention programs that are effective often incorporate group-based components in some way (Conyne & Horne, 2001). The group mode is highly suited for prevention because of its economic advantage over individual approaches, and its capacities for transmitting knowledge, developing competencies, and stimulating direct interaction among participants. These elements are all essential ingredients in successful prevention programs.

Early and focused group interventions have shown success (e.g., Brand, Lakey, & Berman, 1995) in limiting both chronic and severe mental health symptoms, in enhancing the functioning and strengths of participants, and in preventing certain educational and mental health problems. Groups for prevention afford a major step in equalizing and enhancing mental health care (Conyne & Hage, in press).

Prevention groups typically involve small numbers of members who are healthy and/or at risk, and who meet face to face with a trained group leader (or leaders). Members interact with each other. Leaders facilitate an appropriate blend of content (e.g., substance abuse information) with group process (e.g., interpersonal feedback) in order to help members acquire or broaden strengths they can apply to avoid future harmful events and situations and to live their lives more fully (Conyne & Horne, 2001; Conyne & Wilson, 2000). Small psychoeducation groups (Brown, 2008) structured around human relations and skill development hold much promise for reaching prevention goals (DeLucia-Waack, 2006; Ettin, Heiman, & Kopel, 1988; Shechtman, 2001).

Research and Evaluation: "The Proof Is in the Prevention"

"The proof is in the pudding" is another old maxim that Mom (or Dad) might have taught us. It suggests that ingredients, recipes, preparation, equipment, and the cook's skill all affect the pudding but the test of its goodness—the proof—is determined by the pudding itself. Does it work? Will anyone come back for seconds? If you really like it, can you somehow replicate it yourself?

Likewise, "the proof is in the prevention" for prevention programs. Assessment, design, and delivery are all important and each influences a prevention program, but the test of its effectiveness—the proof—is determined by the prevention effect.

Does the prevention program work? Is it effective in promoting well-being and forestalling dysfunction and problems? Can it be replicated, or authentically modified, with other populations and in other settings?

A number of meta-analyses of prevention have been conducted. These studies have identified evidence-based best practices in delivering prevention interventions, which we will turn to in just a moment.

First, though, let me unpack the preceding sentence because it is loaded with complicated terminology. The term *meta-analyses* refers to sets of different statistical techniques that are used to retrieve, select, analyze, and combine research results from related independent studies that have been conducted and reported previously. Thus, an overarching, integrative perspective is yielded that can aid understanding and future progress. *Evidence-based practices* integrate the best research available with acceptable clinical proficiency while factoring in patient characteristics, preferences, and culture (American Psychological Association Presidential Task Force on Evidence-Based Practice, 2006). And *best practices* (which were discussed in Chapter 2) are those that a body of respected colleagues and professional associations have identified as genuinely representing effective and ethical delivery and that can be generalized to comparable situations.

Back to examples of meta-analyses that have been reported in prevention. Dryfoos (2000) reviewed over 100 prevention programs in the areas of school dropout, teen pregnancy, juvenile delinquency, and substance abuse. School-based curricula have been examined (Elias, Gager, & Leon, 1997), as have prevention programs that address children and adolescents (Durlak & Wells, 1997; Weissberg & Greenberg, 1998). Tobler et al. (2000) reported a meta-analysis of 207 universally school-based programs in the area of drug prevention, following such previous analyses by Tobler. Bruvold (1993) presented results of a meta-analysis of adolescent smoking prevention programs. Nation et al. (2003) reported a "review of reviews" that focused on universal and selective prevention programs meeting acceptance criteria in the areas of substance abuse, risky sexual behavior, school failure, and juvenile delinquency and violence. These meta-analyses have contributed to a deeper understanding of the basic tenets of prevention.

Determining prevention effect, though, is much easier said than done. The taste and relative cost of pudding determines its judged value. While arriving at this judgment is subjective, it is pretty straightforward. Taste it—how do you like it? With prevention (or any other mental health or education approach), there is no such simple and direct judgment available, as we somewhat painfully realize. Rather, a set of research and evaluation criteria exist to help arrive at proof.

Those interested in developing and conducting prevention programs will be pleased to discover that an impressive number of programs have been evaluated as being effective, using stringent evaluation criteria to arrive at that judgment. Moreover, resources have been compiled for identifying many of these evidence-based prevention practices, including easily accessible online resources. These resources provide a gateway to effective programs, although the programs contained are not funded well and are not yet being converted to broader application (Dodge, 2008)—but that is another, albeit very important, issue. Nonetheless, guidance is available through these references to assist in program development, implementation, and evaluation. Let's take a look at some of the online resources (Note: See Appendix H for more listings).

Online Resources

An existing, tested program may generally mesh well with local needs or, more likely, might provide the scaffolding for careful adaptation. Another way of saying this is that it may not be necessary to "reinvent the wheel" in many cases (although in some situations creative innovation is necessary or desirable). Regardless, though, when planning a prevention effort, it is advisable to carefully review resources containing evidence-based programs for input (see Byrd & Reininger, 2009, and Conyne, 2004, for two helpful compilations).

For instance, Byrd and Reininger (2009) summarize 36 online resources that list and describe evidence-based prevention programs, and I encourage you to access this source. As an introduction to online resources, 5 of them are extracted here:

1. Agency for Healthcare Research and Quality (AHRQ; http://www.ahrq.gov): Clicking on "Evidence-Based Practice" ushers you into an identification of effective prevention programs based on rigorous scientific analyses. Although many of the examples are more clinically focused, public health prevention programs also are included.

2. Center for Study and Prevention of Violence (CSPV, 1996; http://www .colorado.edu/cspv): Its "Blueprints" and "CSPV Databases" sections provide interactive, searchable databases of effective prevention interventions in violence and other related subjects. Model programs (n = 11) meeting strict criteria for scientific evidence are listed, and another 18 promising programs are identified.

3. The Collaborative for Academic, Social, and Emotional Learning (http://www.casel.org): This registry lists effective prevention programs that promote social and emotional learning in schools, as well as others that have not yet met the "select" criteria used in the evaluation process.

4. The Guide to Community Services (http://www.thecommunityguide.org): This Web site of the Centers for Disease Control and Prevention provides review results on the effectiveness and cost effectiveness of fundamental community preventive health services.

5. National Registry of Evidence-Based Programs and Practices (http://www .nrepp.samhsa.gov): This Web site of the Substance Abuse and Mental Health Services Administration features model programs that have evidenced solid proof of preventing or reducing substance abuse and other high-risk behaviors in schools, communities, and work settings.

Evidence-Based Criteria

What means were used to judge programs deemed to be effective? In the Colorado Blueprints project, for example, the criteria used are that the program showed evidence of (a) a deterrent effect within a strong research design; (b) sustained effects that endure for at least 1 year beyond the prevention program's completion; (c) multiple-site replication, demonstrating that the principles and processes of the program are not limited to one setting alone; and (d) important mediating effects being addressed (e.g., risk and protective factors), as well as the program being cost effective.

Criteria used in other evidence-based examinations, such as by the National Registry of Evidence-Based Programs and Practices, are similarly strict. Notable minimum requirements are that the preventive intervention is able to demonstrate one or more positive outcomes, results have been published in a peer-review publication or have been specified in an evaluation report, and the public can access intervention documentation. Extra points are earned when a quasi-experimental or experimental research design was employed.

Common Denominators of Successful Programs

In addition to evidence-based criteria, which tend to address outcomes and how they were achieved, other important criteria focus more directly on the programs themselves. The following material is adapted from Conyne (2004):

14 Ounces of Prevention. Price, Cowen, Lorion, and Ramos-McKay (1988) identified five "common denominators of success" that applied to the primary prevention programs that were idefntified as "excellent" in the 14 Ounces of Prevention study. These programs

  (a) were targeted and well planned, containing multiple components that were sensitive to the population and setting as well as to the conditions to be prevented;
  (b) were designed to positively alter the life trajectories of participants, that is, to change future patterns of behavior, life conditions, and social settings;
  (c) provided new skills and social support so that program participants gain resources and repertoires in such areas as communication and problem solving that can make a positive difference in their lives;
  (d) strengthened natural support systems, parsimoniously accentuating positive processes that already exist rather than importing more costly external resources; and
  (e) were able to demonstrate evidence of success in terms of reduced occurrence of problems and in strengthened functioning.

Criteria to Assess Programming. Durlak (2003) suggests eight generalizations that characterize effective prevention and health promotion programming. It is reassuring that these points are highly consistent with those presented by Price et al., above, and with some of the evidence-based criteria, suggesting that general agreement about evaluative criteria exists. You will recognize some of these criteria from earlier in this chapter.

According to Durlak, successful prevention and health promotion programming interventions (a) are data based and theory driven, (b) recognize that adjustment is affected by multiple factors at multiple levels, (c) emphasize behavior change and skill development, (d) are well timed, (e) use developmentally appropriate techniques and materials, (f) monitor to assure good program implementation, (g) are tailored and adapted for the particular population and setting, and (h) are evaluated carefully.

When I teach students in my graduate level Preventive Counseling course how to analyze preventive interventions, I provide them with criteria to use in describing and evaluating the programs. These criteria were constructed to subsume those presented by Price et al. and Durlak, and to be consistent with evidence-based approaches. The resulting 47 criteria, arranged into eight categories (purpose; population; methods and settings; timing and appropriateness; personal competencies; system-centered changes; role; and planning, research, and evaluation) are presented next (expanded from Conyne, 2004).

A Checklist of Criteria for Evaluating Prevention Programs

Purposes

- ☐ What is being prevented or promoted?
- ☐ What is the program's purposive strategy (system change, person change, everyday prevention)?
- ☐ What are the program goals and objectives?
- ☐ How do they relate to methods?

Population

- ☐ What is the target population?
- ☐ How are the program participants functioning (well functioning, at risk, early stage of problem)?

Methods and Settings

- ☐ How is assessment involved?
- ☐ How have evidence-based methods been considered and/or used?
- ☐ What methods of intervention are used (education, organization, media, consultation, advocacy, intended prevention within remedial methods, etc.)?
- ☐ Is multiplicity addressed through components, levels, methods?
- ☐ How are setting members involved in the program phases?
- ☐ What settings are involved (family, work, school, neighborhood, other)?
- ☐ How are person-centered and system-centered variables included?
- ☐ How do methods and settings interact?
- ☐ How do they relate to program purposes?
- ☐ How is the program adapted culturally?
- ☐ How are social justice values incorporated?

Timing and Appropriateness

- ☐ How is the program timed (before the fact, early stage)?
- ☐ How is developmental and contextual appropriateness addressed?

Gradients

☐ How is the gradient of Stressors + Organic Factors + Exploitation/Self-Esteem + Coping Skills + Support involved?
☐ How is the gradient of Risk Factors/Protective Factors involved?

Personal Competencies

☐ How is knowledge developed?
☐ How are skills developed?
☐ How are values and attitudes addressed?

System-Centered Changes

☐ How is social support incorporated?
☐ How are environmental factors addressed?
☐ How are stressors reduced?
☐ How are oppression and exploitation addressed (if a factor)?

Role

☐ What is the program deliverer's role or roles (e.g., direct service counselor, researcher, director, group facilitator, consultant, evaluator)?
☐ To what degree is collaboration manifested?

Planning, Research, and Evaluation

☐ To what degree are program development and evaluation steps represented in the program?
☐ Does evaluation address both process and outcome?
☐ Can core components of the program be identified?
☐ How has the program been adapted?
☐ Is the program culturally relevant or potentially culturally relevant?
☐ To what degree is collaboration with participants evidenced?
☐ Does the program include direct, interactive experience?
☐ How sophisticated is the research design?
☐ How contextually sensitive is the research design?
☐ Are results evidence based?
☐ Are results documented?
☐ Are results sustainable?
☐ Have results been published?
☐ Have results been otherwise disseminated?
☐ Have results been replicated?
☐ Has the program been tested across settings?
☐ Is the program cost effective?

In addition to using these criteria to analyze existing prevention programs, they can serve as a checklist to assist program development.

LEARNING EXERCISE **3.1**

Applying Prevention
Criteria to a Model Program

Let's try to summarize your learning at this point. You've been reading about several criteria that are useful for assessing prevention programs and that also are helpful to keep in mind when designing such programs. Choose ONE of these criteria and apply it to the following description of the Life Skills Training (LST) program of Botvin and colleagues (from the Blueprints project):

Program Targets: LST targets all middle/junior high school students, with booster sessions occurring in the 2 years following program completion.

Program Content: LST is intended to prevent or reduce gateway drug use (i.e., tobacco, alcohol, and marijuana). The 3-year program is primarily implemented in school classrooms by school teachers. LST is delivered in 15 sessions in year 1, 10 sessions in year 2, and 5 sessions in year 3. Sessions last an average of 45 minutes and can be delivered once a week or as an intensive mini-course. The program consists of three major elements: (a) general self-management skills, (b) social skills, and (c) information and skills specifically related to drug use. Skills are learned through the use of training techniques such as instruction, demonstration, feedback, reinforcement, and practice.

What did you discover when doing this exercise?

Hey! We Can't Do Everything:
The Ethic and Importance of Collaboration

Indeed, there is no way that any one professional or professional organization (such as a counseling center) can be expected to deliver in all these areas. Each of us possesses our own areas of expertise, and for most of us, these are limited and focused. That's only the way it should be. Being ethical practitioners, our job is to identify and function within our areas of expertise and to know when, where, and how to refer to or to collaborate with others whose expertise is found in other needed areas.

There really is no predicament here but, rather, an opportunity. What is it? The opportunity is the gift of collaboration. After all, prevention is a team-based, interdependent activity where professionals function together and with members of an identified population to produce a workable prevention plan that can be effectively delivered and evaluated.

Diverse competencies, experience levels, and perspectives are melded into a team as prevention is undertaken. Embracing and enacting such a collaborative spirit is a prevention ethic to be cultivated.

Collaboration to pool expertise and experience can occur in two ways. First, a team can be formed to produce or to adapt a new prevention program. This is the strategy that is focused on in this book. In the second case, two or more partner organizations, each owning a successful track record in their own area, can combine their respective resources to yield an adapted prevention effort. An example includes grafting a mental health component to the root of an already successful community sports or arts program so that intentional attention is given to psychological or educational goals.

See what you can do with the following learning exercise that considers collaboration.

LEARNING EXERCISE 3.2

Forming a Collaboration

A. Write your thoughts to the following three questions:

   1. What skills does it take to work well collaboratively?
   2. How can a staff member of a counseling agency function in this way?
   3. Indeed, how can a counseling agency itself do so?

B. Imagine that your counseling agency is interested in preventing high school dropouts in your community. Thinking collaboratively, what general strategies might be possible to pursue?

Developing an understanding of prevention criteria can aid in both the evaluation of preventive programs and their creation. So, spending time learning and applying them will enhance your effectiveness in prevention program development and evaluation.

Summary

Just what constitutes prevention and how to determine whether a program is credible can be difficult tasks. How to create prevention programs can also be an uncertain proposition: Where do you begin? This chapter sought to address these issues by focusing on prevention criteria—those elements that can help define what prevention is, whether a program might be successful, and how to develop programming.

The main criteria for judging and creating prevention programs that were discussed in this chapter include: (a) comprehensiveness, (b) direct experiencing, (c) sufficient dosage, (d) theory driven, (e) provide opportunities for positive relationships, (f) appropriately timed, (g) sociocultural relevance, (h) competent staff, (i) readiness of setting, (j) involvement of effective collaborative community partnerships, (k) delivered with fidelity and with fit, and (l) use of groups.

Research and evaluation also was considered as it relates to criteria. Results of meta-analyses were summarized, several online resources were identified that point to evidence-based programs, common denominators of program success were enumerated, and an extensive checklist for assessing prevention programs was presented.

Finally, the ethic of collaboration in prevention programming was highlighted as essential to good practice. There is no realistic way that any one professional or professional organization can do everything. We all need to work together in sharing resources, experience, and perspectives in planning and delivering prevention programs. Creative and resource-rich programs can result.

CHAPTER 4

Reducing Incidence in Prevention

Chapter Overview

- Why Incidence Reduction?
- Incidence Reduction Formulae for Prevention Planning
- Learning Exercise 4.1. Determining Incidence
- The Adapted and Expanded Albee Incidence Reduction Formula
- Learning Exercise 4.2. Thinking About Decreasing Deficits
- Learning Exercise 4.3. Building a Stronger Social Circle
- Learning Exercise 4.4. Becoming a Strengths-Based Advocate
- Summary

Why Incidence Reduction?

A famous fable exists in the field of prevention. It goes something like the following, adapted from Rappaport (1972):

> You're lolling about on a beautiful afternoon along the bank of a quickly moving stream. Dozing on a blanket you suddenly awake to the sound of shouts. Someone has fallen in the water upstream and is being swept downward by the flow. Alarmed, you dive in at some risk and pull the person safely to shore. Relieved, you return to your blanket, only to find it necessary to rescue another, and then yet another who fall into the fast-moving water. Worn out, you pick up your blanket and go home, satisfied that you were able to help, but very tired.

This fable contains a prevention message. What is it?

Two words: incidence reduction.

Saving people from drowning is noble and important, and it can get to be exhausting. Preventing them from falling into the water in the first place, let's say by building a fence or teaching them how to swim are preferred strategies. Why? They prevent new problems by stopping them from occurring. That is the essence of incidence reduction.

A close consideration of the incidence of a problem is needed. That is the focus of this chapter. You will recall that incidence of a problem refers to the number or the rate of new cases developing, for example, the new cases of suicide, substance abuse, interpersonal violence, school dropout, and so on.

Incidence Reduction Formulae for Prevention Planning

The original incidence formula was developed by Albee (1982, 1985) and elaborated by Albee and Gullotta (1997). Albee's formula, which is discussed in more detail later in this chapter, provides the nucleus for understanding prevention today and is expressed as

$$\text{Incidence Reduction} = \frac{\text{Decrease: (Organic Factors} + \text{Stress} + \text{Exploitation)}}{\text{Increase: (Self-Esteem} + \text{Coping Skills} + \text{Support Groups)}}$$

Perhaps the forerunner for Albee's formula can be traced to Kurt Lewin's (1936) conceptualization that Behavior = f(Person × Environment), or B = f(P × E).

As pointed out by Swensen (1968), Pascal (1959) expanded and adapted Lewin's formula, as follows (Note: The term *psychophylaxis* means resistance to stress):

$$\text{Psychological Deficit} = f\left(\frac{\text{Stress, Maladaptive Habits, and Defenses}}{\text{Psychophylaxis, Environmental Support}}\right)$$

Swensen (1968) later adapted Pascal's basic formula for use in case conceptualization, as follows:

$$\text{Deviant Behavior} = f\left(\frac{\text{Stress, Maladaptive Habits, and Defenses}}{\text{Support, Strengths, Adaptive Habits, and Defenses}}\right)$$

Other variations of Albee's basic incidence reduction formula have been created, with some giving more credence to environmental factors. For instance, Elias and Branden (1988) presented a version first developed by Elias that emphasizes risk and protective processes that are focused on the environment. Risk factors in that formula include environmental stressors and related contributors such as economic and financial pressures, while protective factors are defined as socialization practices, social support resources, and opportunities for connectedness.

Bloom (1996) presented a "configural" equation organizing six factors he says need to be considered to optimize effective preventive interventions. Similar to Albee's formula, this framework asks that planners analyze dynamic relationships between the strengths and limitations of people, social supports and stressors, and physical environment resources and pressures.

The formula to be used in this book is an adaptation of Albee's original incidence reduction formula. The adaptation was created by Conyne (see Conyne & Newmeyer, 2008; Conyne, Newmeyer, & Kitchens, 2007) and then further refined. Its value is found in its comprehensiveness and the translation of important deficit and strength factors into concrete planning steps. The incidence reduction approach to prevention program development and evaluation is particularly beneficial at the step of problem identification, because its use allows programs to be shaped intentionally to avoid future occurrences.

These formulae provide frameworks for organizing a comprehensive array of factors that contribute to problem incidence. The programmatic goal is to reduce deficits while increasing strengths. The approaches include elements in the numerator (i.e., those above the line) that represent *deficits,* and elements in the denominator (i.e., those below the line) that represent *strengths.*

Albee's Original Incidence Reduction Formula

Let's now focus on Albee's original approach, which I am repeating below:

Original Albee Incidence Reduction Formula

Decrease:	(Organic Factors + Stress + Exploitation)
Increase:	(Self-Esteem + Coping Skills + Support Groups)

Underlying Concepts. This formula set the stage for identifying problems in terms of avoiding their reoccurrence and then designing programs that might allow this goal to occur. It is a significant framework because it pulled together factors that, although they were known to be important for prevention, had not yet been linked coherently.

Note that essential organizing concepts are embedded in the formula. First, it suggests an ecological approach. Elements included in the numerator, referring to deficits, trace their origin to the environment (E). On the other hand, elements included in the denominator of the formula, referring to strengths, trace their origin to persons (P) and relationships. In this conception, personal elements are important but not enough. Effects of the environment, such as sources of stress, also need to be considered. This was an important contribution.

The Albee formula (Albee, 1982) suggests that these environmental and personal elements exist and need to be considered in dynamic relationship—that is, they interact. Prevention programs, then, need to be designed and conducted to reflect this interaction. How to do this? Reduce the intensity of the deficits while increasing the force of the strengths.

This approach captures the contributions of a legend to planned social psychology, group dynamics, and planned social change, Kurt Lewin. Among other innovations, Lewin (1936) suggested the ecological concept that behavior is a function of persons interacting with their environment (B = f[P × E]). He also developed a widely used social change technique, force field analysis (FFA; 1943). In FFA, driving and restraining forces in a field (or dynamic environment, such as a classroom) are analyzed in an effort to produce intentional strategies to reduce effects of the blocks, to enhance effects of the supports, and ultimately to alter the equilibrium of the field to a more positive state.

These fundamental concepts can be used by prevention planners to help in identifying potential problem areas and then to move ahead with designing prevention programs. Below we will begin to examine aspects of the Albee incidence formula.

Deficit Elements in the Numerator of the Formula: Decrease Organic Factors + Stress + Exploitation. Albee packed a lot of wisdom into the elements of his formula. For the numerator (deficits, largely environmental), he identified environmental contributions to organic dysfunction, sources of stress, and forces for exploitation existing in the environment.

Organic factors in Albee's conception did not focus on internal, biological causes. Although substantial and exciting advancements are occurring through genetic research today (e.g., the capacity to learn about one's genotype, with preventive implications galore), Albee focused on environmental causes of organic dysfunction. He thought these were what psychologists, counselors, social workers, and policy makers could influence through research and advocacy.

Examples include how physical and mental functioning can be impaired through the abuse of chemical substances, the effects of lead-based paint, and the consequences of infectious diseases. Causes of autism are thought to be both genetic and environmental. With the latter, such environmental factors as toxins, chemicals, pesticides, flame retardants, and pre- and postnatal viruses may all play a role. In the case of obesity, although internal biological causes exist, the environment also exerts strong effects. Simply consider the physical layout of many neighborhoods, with sidewalks and green spaces lacking, with the result that regular physical exercise is inconvenient and sometimes dangerous.

Stress is an omnipresent companion in everyday life. As Selye (1974) pointed out, stress can be salutary (positive) and it can be pathogenic (negative). He termed these two possibilities "eustress" and distress, respectively. Here is an example of the difference. Tomorrow evening I am scheduled to present the keynote address at a conference. This event is a potential source of either eustress or of distress for me. If I allow its importance to become excessive, leading to a high amount of anxiety, I am susceptible to generating too much stress and doing poorly. Conversely, if I am able to keep the event "in check," where some but not too much anxiety is generated, this lowered amount of stress might serve to nudge me forward to perform well, all things considered. The point here is that stress is not necessarily a negative condition. Rather, it is a fact of life and can promote or detract from enjoyment, satisfaction, and productivity.

By any stretch, however, distress plays a corrosive role in daily life, with various studies linking it with a range of physical diseases and psychological dysfunctions. Distress, therefore, is noxious and it is a major contemporary problem.

Events such as the speech I mentioned can be thought of as an everyday "stressor." They arise from the environment. Our reactions to them are what constitute stress and its impact. So there is much that people can do to moderate their stress levels. These actions are considered in the denominator of Albee's equation, which will be considered shortly.

At the same time, though, modern life is fast paced and demanding. Many stressors (sources of stress) are largely or totally out of our personal control and influence. A difficult economy with rising unemployment, falling wages, and increasing costs conspires to yield challenges that are excessive for many. Eighty percent of American adults report the economy being a significant source of stress in 2008, with higher numbers of women than men being affected (American Psychological Association, 2008c). A cyclone, tornado, earthquake, flood, or other natural disaster can swoop in unexpectedly, leaving in its path chaos, destruction, and mayhem. Terrorist and mass murder attacks that are becoming all too familiar constitute a type of human-caused disaster that shocks and traumatizes.

Other stressors may be controllable, to some degree. Ongoing stressful life events, such as time demands, boring tasks, fear of unemployment, giving a speech, and traffic jams, can nag and bite at you. Prevention seeks to remove the negative stressors or to diminish their potential impact through before-the-fact skill-building programs. By doing so, the corrosive force on people is eased or eliminated, leading to the possibility of less stress being experienced.

Exploitation occurs when a person takes advantage of someone else, either intentionally or unintentionally. Albee's inclusion of exploitation as a source of deficits was significant. All the societal "isms" represent sources of exploitation: ageism, sexism, racism, classism, to name a few, and these often result in marginalization of those exploited.

Two acronyms, ADDRESSING (Hays, 1996) and RESPECTFUL (D'Andrea & Daniels, 2001), serve to organize many demographic and cultural factors that, when abused, contribute to exploitation and oppression. These are listed below:

ADDRESSING issues:

Age/generational factors

Developmental or acquired Disabilities

Religion and spiritual orientation

Ethnicity

Socioeconomic status

Sexual orientation

Indigenous heritage

National origin

Gender

RESPECTFUL issues:

Religious/spiritual

Economic class

Sexual identity

Psychological/developmental

Ethnic/racial identity

Chronological

Trauma and threats to well-being

Family

Unique physical

Language and location of residence

Albee called on preventionists to help produce a "just society" (Albee, 1986) where such factors as sexism, racism, consumerism, ageism, patriarchy, and homophobia are all reduced or eliminated. Taking these steps, he suggested, would lead to a more humane and fair society with positive effects on larger numbers of people who are now too frequently exploited and out of the mainstream.

Social justice is a major goal for prevention (Kenny et al., 2009; Prilleltensky & Nelson, 1997), and vice versa. Personal and environmental approaches to prevention can be geared toward advancing strengths and to lowering or obliterating exploitation. They take differing routes, with the environmental track often targeting public policy changes or client advocacy within the legislative or legal system (Vera, Buhin, & Isacco, 2009).

Strengths-Based Elements in the Denominator of the Formula: Increase Self-Esteem + Coping Skills + Support Groups. A "strengths-based approach" to counseling is receiving increased importance today (e.g., Aspinall & Staudinger, 2003; E. Smith, 2006), including the exploding amount of work in positive psychology (e.g., Snyder & Lopez, 2002). This approach seeks to help clients to become aware of, and to employ, existing assets. It contrasts with, and can be integrated with, a deficits approach where identification of dysfunctions takes precedence. Too often clients (and their counselors) overlook natural strengths, whether these be interests, abilities, values, attitudes, or experience—while being hypersensitive to their inadequacies and problems. This negative tilt leads to a misrepresentation of their capacities. A strengths-based approach shares much in common with positive psychology (e.g., Peterson & Seligman, 2004), and with the bedrock foundation of the counseling and counseling psychology professions (e.g., Kaczmarek, 2006).

Albee developed his model decades before the contemporary attention being given to strengths-based practice. He thought it was important to examine and address both deficits and strengths, both risk factors and protective factors, to use related terminology. The denominator of his formula organized these factors into three categories: (a) self-esteem, (b) coping skills, and (c) support groups.

Self-esteem refers to a relatively stable sense of one's own self-worth, self-regard, and self-respect. Self-esteem can be thought of as the emotional component of self-concept. A realistic and positive self-esteem is important to a healthy life.

Since the 1980s, when Albee included self-esteem in his formula, the understanding of the concept and its overall role in healthy functioning has been met with a certain degree of controversy. Some research seems to indicate that high self-esteem is not necessarily associated with healthy functioning, and in some cases where unearned high levels of self-esteem exist, it may be associated with negative behaviors, such as bullying or other forms of violence. An aggressive focus on developing self-esteem has been found by some critics to exert too much emphasis on the self, smacking of narcissism (Baumeister, Smart, & Boden, 1996). Seligman (2002a) adds that the "self-esteem movement" of the 1970s, with its "feel-good ethic" (p. 217), may have contributed unintentionally to low self-esteem on a massive scale.

Self-esteem does not mean cheap success or a life without challenge. It is a vital component of a satisfying life. Intentional attention in prevention programs to buttress a realistic sense of self-esteem while attending to other areas as well, such as increased social connection, is a desirable ingredient of positive mental health. Therefore, when identifying and assessing problems, detecting the presence of self-esteem in a population is a vital step to take.

Coping skills are the tools people use to negotiate life challenges and stressful situations. Coping skills may help a person confront a situation, take action, and move ahead, while remaining flexible and persistent in solving problems. Proactive coping (Schwarzer & Knoll, 2003) moves the coping bar higher, dealing with how people master challenging demands, prepare for uncertain events, and search for meaning. *The Proactive Coping Inventory* (Greenglass, Schwarzer, & Taubert, 1999) provides a 14-item assessment of this concept.

People can be helped to develop coping skills through prevention programs. Examples of such coping skills (sometimes termed *life skills*) include: decision making, problem solving, anticipating and managing anxiety, stress management, social skills (communication, forming friendships, relating effectively with those one is attracted to, being assertive), initiating activities, collaborating with others, finding and giving support, and more. These kinds of competencies are generally useful and can be adapted across a wide range of situations and events (Botvin & Tortu, 1988; Danish & Forneris, 2006).

Support groups refer to informal, primary, and face-to-face involvements with family and friends that convey a buffering and protective effect against life stressors. They also refer to intentionally formed associations such as clubs and organizations, and to groups formed specifically for support and psychological assistance.

Regarding the first type of support group, you may recall the Ruby and Oren Principle I wrote of earlier, where they derived so much benefit from their decades-long Saturday afternoon card game with close friends. Involvement with clubs and organizations, religious settings, volunteer efforts, and other more formalized means of association characterize the second form. In the third way toward social support, people can become part of counseling or therapy groups and of the thousands of support groups that exist across the country for a wide variety of problems and issues.

So this is the classic formulation of incidence reduction in prevention. The number or the rate of development of new cases of a disorder can be lowered through prevention programs that cut the negative impact of environmental factors (numerator), by those that boost the effect of positive factors (denominator), or through those programs that accomplish both simultaneously. Next we will examine the adaptation of that formula that will be followed throughout this book to tailor problem identification with program development.

LEARNING EXERCISE 4.1

Determining Incidence

Suppose the existing percentage of students who failed to graduate from Jackson High School was 19% in 2007. As a school counselor there, you created a team of staff, parents, and students whose main goal was to lower the incidence of academic failure and to increase the graduation rate beginning with 2009. Circle below which percentage rate would reflect reduction of incidence in the failure rate, and then explain why.

   a. 16%

   b. 19%

   c. 22%

The Adapted and Expanded Albee Incidence Reduction Formula

General Version

Incidence Reduction Formula for Problem Identification in Prevention Program Development and Evaluation

---

Decrease: DEFICITS
              Environmental Risks and Stressors: (Physical $\times$ Social $\times$ Culture)

Increase: STRENGTHS
              Protective Factors: (Personal $\times$ Interpersonal $\times$ Group $\times$ System)

This adapted and expanded formula for incidence reduction is an attempt to update and to further specify the essential factors Albee identified in his original formula. As mentioned, this version will be used in the prevention program development and evaluation approach to be detailed in subsequent chapters.

Underlying Conceptual Changes in the Adapted Formula

Carrying forward the earlier discussion of Albee's formula, the adapted version continues a focus on lowering negative environmental factors and increasing positive personal factors. The basic conceptual underpinnings and structure of the original formula are largely retained but are expanded.

The first expansion is tied to a perspective of how deficits and strengths are conceptualized, that is, across a broad scope ranging from individual through global influences. Two other changes are structural in nature and are reflected concretely in the adapted formula: (a) the multiplicative, rather than additive, relationship of factors; and (b) the expansion and specification of factors that are included. These expansions are explained in more detail to follow.

Perspective to be Applied: Wide Scope of Deficits and Strengths

People do not exist in a vacuum. Rather, they live in contexts where ongoing and reciprocal People × Environment interactions occur. These contexts can be proximal (i.e., close by, as in a nuclear family or a work group) or distal (i.e., far away, as in the fall of the Japanese stock market or in a hurricane forming thousands of miles away). Therefore, although not specified concretely in the adapted formula, the scope of deficits and strengths can best be thought of as incorporating a full range of individual to global influences.

This range of scope is drawn from an ecological consideration that was explicated by Bronfenbrenner (1979) and that has been adopted, adapted, and expanded by many others; for instance, it forms the basis of ecological counseling (Conyne & Cook, 2004).

An ecological viewpoint recognizes that persons interact with levels of their environment (Conyne & Clack, 1981; Lewin, 1936; Neufeld et al., 2006). In such a view, individuals are influenced by (and influence) multiple levels of systems. There are many ways to describe these systemic levels. Bronfenbrenner (e.g., 1979) named four successively broader levels of systems:

- Microsystem: primary, face-to-face, ongoing relationships, such as with family;
- Mesosystem: connections between microsystems, such as between home and work;
- Exosystem: larger, but remote systems that affect us, such as health care and government; and
- Macrosystem: cultural, political, and economic "blueprints" that surround and affect us, such as conceptions of the "American Dream" or perhaps what it means to be a man or a woman in our society.

Kasambira and Edwards (2000) and Maton (2000) proposed that a level be added beyond the macrosystem, seeking to represent "global" and "world" influences, respectively. Other ecological conceptions have been produced, too, including that of the World Health Organization (2002), which places the individual in interaction with relationships, community, and society.

Back to the Expanded Formula

It is recommended that planners take a broad perspective when considering levels and elements contained in the adapted formula's numerator (deficits) and denominator (strengths). Although not all may be pertinent at any one point, these systemic and interactive levels include:

(a) natural and built environment
(b) family, friends, and colleagues
(c) home, school, work, and recreation
(d) neighborhood, community, state, and nation
(e) cultural, political, health, economic, and other policies
(f) macro "blueprints," including culture, gender, ethnicity, race, nationalism, and so on
(g) global and world factors

Basic Structural Change One: Multiplicative Effect of Factors in Numerator and Denominator

This structural change recognizes that influencing effects are more than additive. Rather than A + B + C, the situation in real life is actually A × B × C. Our lives are mutually influenced and interactive, not linear and static. For instance, how the pressure of an economic downturn combines with divorce proceedings is untold by attempting to add up separate units of distress. Here, we need to go to the multiplication table, instead, because effects build on each other, reverberating and recycling, combining and shifting, to yield forces exceeding results obtained by independent analysis alone. Indeed, the whole is much larger than the sum of its parts.

Basic Structural Change Two: Expansion and specification of factors included in the version below, which is useful for prevention program planning, especially for problem identification.

Decrease: DEFICITS

Environmental Risks and Stressors: (Physical × Social × Culture)
Physical Environment: Stressors in Natural and Built Environment
Social Environment: Stressors in Informal and Formal Social Relations
Culture: Exploitation, Oppression, Underlying Values and Patterns

Increase: STRENGTHS

Protective Factors: (Personal × Interpersonal × Group × System)
Personal Factors: Self-Esteem, Well-Being, Resilience, Self-Efficacy
Interpersonal Factors: Interpersonal and Coping Skills, Engagement
Group Factors: Collective Efficacy, Social Support
System Factors: Ecological Competence, Advocacy

You will notice right away that the adapted formula contains more factors that are organized under revised titles of "environmental deficits" (numerator) and "personal, interpersonal, and group strengths" (denominator). The retitling and expansion are intended to reflect advancements in research and practice that have occurred since Albee's original formulation. These adaptations will be addressed in the next two sections, dealing with decreasing deficits and increasing strengths.

Deficit-Based Elements in the Adapted Formula

Consistent with Albee's viewpoint, deficits are presented in the numerator of the formula. These are environmental factors, which, theoretically at least, can be influenced through environmentally centered preventive approaches. One example, considering organic deficits, is to eliminate exposure of children to lead in paint and other substances in an effort to reduce lead poisoning. Although significant innovations are occurring—and will continue to appear—in genome and related biologically oriented investigations, practice and ethics have not yet caught up with science.

Most environmentally centered preventive efforts involve assessing and developing programs that target stressors in the physical and social environment, and in the environment's culture. Here, we talk about "stressors," not "stress." This distinction is not simply a matter of semantics. Environmental stressors are potential sources of (dis)stress, which is an experienced state. Distress can result when the strength of the source exceeds a person's capacity to cope effectively and without strain. In prevention, we want to eliminate or decrease the force and power of *sources* of problems.

Environmental stressors can be traced to physical, social, and culture aspects of the environment. The *physical environment* includes both natural and human-made (built) forms. The *social environment* contains informal and naturally occurring interpersonal relations and those that occur through organized settings such as work, school, and neighborhood. *Culture* in this formula refers specifically to values, attitudes, beliefs, and general practices that exploit or oppress others, often—but not necessarily—as an unintended side effect. Prevention programs try to:

Decrease: DEFICITS

Environmental Stressors and Risk Factors:
(Physical × Social × Culture)

Physical Environment: Stressors in Natural and Built Environment

Social Environment: Stressors in Informal and Formal Social Relations

Culture: Exploitation, Oppression, Underlying Values and Patterns

Deficits in the Physical Environment. Here are some isolated examples of deficits in the natural environment. Current world weather patterns frequently devastate populations with excessive, often unpredicted, and deadly strikes involving tornados, hurricanes and cyclones, earthquakes, and other natural calamities. Pandemic viruses threaten to attack. Malaria, tuberculosis, and AIDS run rampant in parts of Africa. Food shortages plague millions around the world.

Following are some examples of deficits in the built environment. Obesity is a serious problem in this country and increasingly around the world. For example, in the last 25 years the number of obese American adults has increased from 14.5% to 32.2%. This is serious not only due to the immediate problems with being obese (e.g., mobility) but even more so due to the heightened risk of suffering diabetes, coronary heart disease, and cancer (Department of Health and Human Services, 2001). In terms of the built environment, many neighborhoods have been constructed that provide no ready means for walking, riding a bike, running, or other forms of physical exercise. Foods available in typical "Mom & Pop" stores in the inner city or in rural villages tend to be non-nutritious and fattening. These deficits can contribute to obesity (Conyne, 2008b).

In other examples of deficits in the built environment, trying to teach using small-group formats becomes inconvenient and complicated because many classrooms contain chairs or desks that are immovable or very difficult to move. Indeed, the concrete and steel construction of many large, public buildings (consider many university residence halls as an example) are largely impervious to human imprint (Sommer, 1974).

In a broader sense, some buildings themselves are "sick." Two forms of building sickness have been identified. Sick building syndrome (SBS) applies to buildings that appear to cause acute illnesses but where no specific cause is found, and building-related illness (BRI) applies where airborne building contaminants have been specifically identified as causing diagnosable diseases (U.S. Environmental Protection Agency, 2008).

Although prevention programs cannot stop natural disasters from occurring, they can be developed to help ready an at-risk population for the eventuality of such events. As well, early intervention programs can be provided following a catastrophe—to listen, offer support, and perhaps refer to therapy in an effort to lessen the time to recovery and the severity of reactions. As American Red Cross Disaster Mental Health volunteers, we sometimes have the tasks of offering preventive education to community groups about potential natural disasters (such as a threatening flu pandemic) and being quickly on the scene providing casualty support following a natural disaster, such as a deadly fire or a destructive tornado.

Deficits in the Social Environment. The social environment is made up of both informal and formal relations. These can be for good or ill, depending on the situation. Informal relations include the availability and strength of everyday interactions with those near us—friends, family, neighbors—and those available to us at longer distance or through electronic means. This can be viewed as our informal "social network."

Formal relations in the social environment include our local and long-distance associations with organized social structures. Examples of these formal settings include work settings, governmental offices, religious institutions, political organizations, and the like. Through these organizations people come into contact with colleagues, staff, consumers, events and experiences, and policies and procedures. These may be thought of as our formal social network.

Next are some illustrations of informal social relations that represent deficits. The thinness of a social network can lead to physical and psychological problems. When few people are available to share life's slings and arrows, as well as its high points, a sense of social isolation can take hold. One consequence is that, when needed, there may be no one to turn to. I recently suffered a sudden tear in the retina of my right eye. My wife was out of town for several days, leaving me alone. While usually this does not pose a problem, when the back of my eye suddenly streaked with blood while I was home alone one evening, I immediately felt the need for support. Fortunately, my daughter lives nearby and my son was returning from college the next day, so help was available. In other examples, social relations can turn ugly and difficult, leading to high states of anxiety. Families can become disrupted through marital discord, or when children experience significant problems at school. Even moving naturally through predictable human developmental stages, such as becoming a teen or moving into retirement, can present challenges in social relations.

In our contemporary, highly technologized life, informal social relations also can occur electronically, as I mentioned, through such social networking spots as Facebook, MySpace, and Twitter. Although these resources certainly can promote positive social connections and communication, as with any resource they also possess the capacity for abuse. For instance, some users can become addicted to electronic social connections, leaving flesh-and-blood interactions behind. Too, these cyberspace methods have been used to bully others. In an extreme cyberbullying case (Keefe, 2008), a 13-year-old girl hanged herself allegedly due to a MySpace relationship that turned very bad with an older woman who had been posing as a 16-year-old boy.

In formal social relations, people interact with others within organized systems that have rules, policies, procedures, resources, and cultures. The nature of interaction is more formally prescribed and usually involves some form of task accomplishment: learning something (e.g., in the classroom), gaining something (e.g., a spiritual experience in a religious setting), producing something (e.g., at work), getting something (e.g., purchasing a product or a service), giving something (e.g., volunteering), and so on. Social relations in such environments sometimes receive lesser priority than task productivity. The culture of an organization sometimes can be oppressive. Occasionally staff can be disrespectful to consumers. At times collegial relations can be dominated by competition and mean-spiritedness. Too often demands on workers exceed resources. In these and other situations, the formal social environment can be an inhospitable place impacting people negatively.

Deficits in the Culture. Every environment is characterized by and through its culture. What are its underlying values and patterns? Is it open or closed? Supportive or competitive? Rigid or flexible? Does it promote growth or constrain it? Of particular importance in prevention is the degree to which any environment's culture suppresses its members or supports and encourages them.

Even more central to this issue is the question of whether the culture reflects values, beliefs, attitudes, and patterns that serve to exploit and oppress those who function in the environment (e.g., staff, consumers) through policies, procedures, and behaviors. Exploitation and oppression are related forces that are of concern to prevention due to the social injustice that results. When a person or group is exploited or oppressed by others, it results in gains for those others and disempowers those who are taken advantage of, resulting in fewer resources, lessened control, disenfranchisement, and emotional and psychological harm.

Exploitation and oppression can be blatant, as in legislation, rules, or policies that disallow reasonable access to services or resources. Being denied the right to vote based on gender, race, or ethnicity is an example drawn from our country's history that was finally corrected. These conditions are usually controversial, with people holding differing points of view. A current debate, involving the right of gays to marry, is one such instance, as is the issue of women being unable to secure the priesthood in certain religious orders.

Exploitation and oppression also can occur in subtle forms, being institutionalized within the policies and practices of an organization, community, or nation. Often this form may be unintentional and unconscious or can be defended by using certain criteria that are frequently economic in nature. For example, the failure to include full-service grocery stores in the urban core perhaps can be explained in bottom-line economic terms, but its effect can be exploitative and oppressive on those who live in that city's section where nutritious food is largely unavailable. The fact that some 47 million citizens are without health insurance in our country can be explained in numerous ways, including the legislation that is in place that makes acquiring such insurance out of reach financially for so many. It can be argued that this situation exploits and oppresses those citizens, leading to undiagnosed and untreated diseases and to elevated societal costs of many kinds.

Program development environmental deficits—physical, social, culture—are important to assess, identify, and evaluate for their effects. This information then becomes central to program design considerations.

LEARNING EXERCISE 4.2

Thinking About Decreasing Deficits

Decreasing deficits is an important incidence reduction goal in prevention programming. Often these deficits are found in the environment: its physical, social, and cultural dimensions. These dimensions can be found all around us, in families, work, school, policies and procedures, the cultural milieu, and events transpiring around the world. For example, severe changes in economic stability exert powerful effects on all of us.

Think about your own environment. What factors are you aware of that affect you?

Jot down those factors. Then organize them into these categories:

Family, education, economy, politics, work, and world

What do you find? What negative factors could potentially be reduced? Make some notes below:

_____

_____

_____

Strengths-Based Elements in the Adapted Formula

Again, consistent with the original formula, the denominator contains strengths-based elements—but more of them, and organized within a broader rubric. Where Albee included self-esteem, coping skills, and support groups, the adapted formula expands this organizing conception to embrace personal, interpersonal, group, and system strengths. Please refer to material in the earlier section related to Albee's formula for a discussion of self-esteem, coping skills, and support groups. Below is a discussion of the broader organizing rubric of personal, interpersonal, group, and system strengths.

Increase: STRENGTHS

Protective Factors: (Personal × Interpersonal × Group × System)

Personal Factors: Self-Esteem, Well-Being, Resilience, Self-Efficacy

Interpersonal Factors: Interpersonal and Coping Skills, Engagement

Group Factors: Collective Efficacy, Social Support

System Factors: Ecological Competence, Advocacy

Personal Strengths (self-esteem, well-being, resilience, self-efficacy). In general, people possess remarkably strong physical and psychological resources. Although we cannot leap tall mountains in single bounds, like Superman, barring disability and poor health we can climb mountains, ford small streams, work long hours, persist over time with grit, develop and maintain meaningful relationships, and much—much—more.

We owe much of this capacity to personal strengths found in self-esteem (previously discussed), well-being, resilience, and self-efficacy. Let's consider the latter three strengths.

Well-Being. Happiness is a part of well-being, and it has assumed both a popular and a scientific following. In the first instance, the quest for happiness is marked by the National Pursuit of Happiness Week during November (Scott, 2008). Popular songs also have drawn our attention to happiness. "Don't Worry, Be Happy" is the title of a bouncy song by Bobby McFerrin (1988), inspired by the words of the Indian spiritual master Meher Baba. Here is one verse from the song: "In your life expect some trouble, but when you worry you make it double. Don't worry, be happy." In another hit song, "Soak Up the Sun," Sheryl Crow (2002) said it this way: "It's not having what you want, it's wanting what you've got." But probably to find the clearest musical theme for well-being and happiness we should turn to the classic advice of Johnny Mercer and Harold Arlen, and sung by Bing Crosby (Mercer & Arlen, 1944) in "Here Come the Waves":

> You've got to accentuate the positive
>
> Eliminate the negative
>
> And latch on to the affirmative
>
> Don't mess with Mr. In-Between.*

This advice, I think, cuts to the quick of well-being and happiness and their place within the scientific study of positive psychology (e.g., Frederickson, 1998; Peterson

*Source: Used with permission. www.johnnymercer.com.

& Seligman, 2004; Snyder & Lopez, 2002, 2007). Adapting an observation by Keyes (2007), in referring to the Mercer and Arlen refrain, we need to: Accentuate the positive (flourish), eliminate the negative (mental disorders), latch on to the affirmative (positivity), and don't mess with mister in-between (languish). Incidentally, Keyes summarized research data from the MacArthur Foundation's Midlife in the United States (MIDUS) survey (Brim, Ryff, & Kessler, 2004) showing that there is much room for growth in the U.S. adult population. About 10% of the population are flourishing, 50% are moderately healthy psychologically, and the remainder are dealing with mental disorders (20%+) or languishing (10%+).

As Lyubomirsky observes (Novotney, 2008), happiness is the holy grail of science, in part because most people around the world report that they want to be happy. She has been involved with her graduate student colleagues (Lyubomirsky, Sousa, & Dickerhoof, 2006) and others in producing innovative research in the area of happiness. These researchers have found that spending less than 10 minutes a day focusing on happy life events can help people to feel happier, with improved life satisfaction. According to these researchers, 40% of happiness is controllable through such activities, with 50% tied to one's genetic set point, and another 10% associated with life circumstances. See Travis (2006) and Snyder and Lopez (2007) for a number of other positive psychology exercises that can be used daily, and that are aimed at improving mental health. For one example, see Learning Exercise 4.3.

LEARNING EXERCISE 4.3

Building a Stronger Social Circle

Several of the life tasks of adults are related to developing a stronger social network. Picture in your mind your social network. Draw four concentric circles. Write "Me" in the middle circle. Write the names of people with whom you are involved on a continuing basis in each circle around "Me." The closer you are to people, then the closer their names should be to the middle circle.

Consider your social circles as you do the following two exercises:

(a) Write down three strategies for how you can maintain relationships with those closest to you while becoming closer to those in more distant circles:

1. _____

2. _____

3. _____

(b) Choose one strategy and write a short action plan of how you might put this strategy into practice during the next month:

_____

_____

_____

_____

Source: Adapted from Snyder & Lopez, 2007, p. 121.

As I mentioned, the pursuit of happiness is one part of well-being, which is a central organizing framework within the study of positive psychology (e.g., Peterson & Seligman, 2004). Well-being can be thought of as happiness plus meaning. Teasing it apart, well-being comprises psychological, social, and emotional components (Snyder & Lopez, 2007):

Psychological well-being: Self-acceptance, personal growth, purpose in life, environmental mastery, autonomy, positive relations with others

Social well-being: Social acceptance, social actualization, social contribution, social coherence, social integration

Emotional well-being: Positive effect, negative effect, life satisfaction, happiness

Positive values and attitudes, strengths, and character also are associated with well-being and are key dimensions within positive psychology. Assessment tools have been created to identify all of these important concepts (Lopez & Snyder, 2003). These include, but are not limited to, *Gallup's Clifton StrengthsFinder, Values in Action—Inventory of Strengths,* and the *Search Institute Profiles of Student Life.* All are available online (Seligman, 2002b).

Resilience. To be resilient is to "bounce back." Technically, resilience is defined as "a class of phenomena characterized by patterns of positive adaptations in the context of significant adversity or risk" (Masten & Reed, 2002, p. 75). The capacity of Viktor Frankl (1959) to withstand his nightmare experience of internment by the Nazis offers a glowing illustration of resiliency. Werner's classic studies (Werner & Smith, 1982, 1992) of 700 children on the island of Kauai between 1955 and 1995 demonstrated that one third of the cohort who were at-risk for academic and social problems were naturally resilient, due to their dispositions and to available external support.

Consistent with other strengths and virtues in positive psychology, resilience is best understood as an ordinary, not an extraordinary, strength. Masten (2001) emphasizes the "power of the ordinary" in resilience in this way:

Resilience does not come from rare and special qualities, but from the magic of ordinary, normative human resources in the minds, brains, and bodies of children, in their families and relationships, and in their communities. (p. 235)

The capacity of people to spring back when faced with enormous odds is impressive, important, assessable, and teachable. It is an important protective factor in human functioning across the life span, for—as sure as the sun comes up in the east and sets in the west—all of us will encounter tribulations and life tests.

Resiliency is frequently overlooked when designing helping programs of any kind. Certainly, program personnel need to keep the concept of resiliency in mind as they assess, create, deliver, and evaluate prevention initiatives. Tapping into this naturally existing reserve presents a potentially powerful source for growth and change.

Self-Efficacy. Self-efficacy (Bandura, 1997) is the belief that a person possesses the capabilities to "organize and execute the courses of action required to produce given attainments" (p. 3). These beliefs contribute to human agency, the capacity to exercise influence and control over events with which a person is confronted. Developing a sense of mastery of life events is a powerful personal strength, indeed. Dusty Baker, manager of the Cincinnati Reds major league baseball team, was describing self-efficacy when he said about his players, "Once you start coming through, you start believing you *can* come through" (Glynn, 2008).

Self-efficacy can be realized and expressed in the full range of life contexts. One can become efficacious in regard to health matters, in school situations, at work, in relationships, in exercising, and in many other situations. The belief generalizes. Indeed, Bandura suggests that people can exercise control over their personal destinies and in national life.

At the root of self-efficacy is an interdependent, transactional perspective. This view is consistent with the ecological orientation we discussed earlier. People become more self-efficacious by developing attitudes and skills allowing them to transact more effectively with environmental influences and situations. They emerge with a perception based on performance that they can be prime movers in their world, a belief that they can make a difference.

Self-efficacy, as other strength elements, can be taught and learned. For instance, a number of cognitive-behavioral programs are based on this principle.

Identifying the degree to which coping skills, self-efficacy, and human agency are present in a group of people for whom a prevention program may be developed should be a part of prevention assessment, design, delivery, and evaluation.

Interpersonal Strengths (interpersonal and coping skills, engagement). Humans are interpersonal beings. We all live with others, work and play with others, learn from others. Our self-concepts and the meaning we derive from life are dependent on the nature of our human relationships.

These interpersonal relationships occur informally. How positive they are is a function of both opportunity (it's difficult to "be interpersonal" when no one is around) and the skills people possess to form, maintain, and learn from these relationships.

Interpersonal and Coping Skills. Possessing the interest and ability to communicate effectively with others is a basis for positive mental health. Satir (1972), the famous family therapist, observed that communication is the single most significant contributor to the kinds of relationships people make, to what happens to themselves, and to the world. In many ways, we become people through our interpersonal relationships, and their quality shapes the kind of people we become.

In order to develop productive interpersonal relationships, it is necessary to possess or to develop at least adequate interpersonal skills. Assessment of these skills can be very useful in developing prevention programs.

The skills themselves, taken independently, seem simple enough. They include:

Attending

Active listening

Showing interest

Behaving genuinely

Showing respect

Demonstrating caring

Clarifying messages

Communicating understanding

Sending clear messages

Being assertive

Disagreeing positively

Managing conflict

Asking questions

Giving information

Connecting thoughts

Linking statements

Self-disclosing

Giving feedback

Being able to integrate these (and other) interpersonal skills into an effective and appropriate style of interacting with others is a more complex task, and it takes some time and practice to develop competence. For some people, all this comes fairly naturally. For others, it is more difficult. Interpersonal skills training can be a helpful preventive program for many people, and a variety of models and methods exist for this purpose in many disciplines such as psychology, communication, business, management, social work, counseling, and education.

Coping skills were discussed in the context of the original formula by Albee. Please refer to that discussion earlier in this chapter.

Engagement. The comedian, actor, and film director Woody Allen is credited with observing that "80% of success is showing up." Yes, being present is important, but the percentage may be inaccurate. Attendance is a necessary precursor, but it can only set the stage for something to occur. There typically is much more to success, however it may be measured, than merely showing up.

Engagement is critically important, as I emphasized early in this book. By engagement, I mean connecting actively with people and events in the situation at hand. Interaction, vital involvement, and active participation are synonymous terms for this kind of connection. Engagement is associated with the concept of *flow* (Csikszentmihalyi, 1990), a state in which people become positively engrossed in their experience, so much so that they can lose track of time.

Moreover, engagement can occur over time. Persistence supplies the longer-term commitment that allows engagement to be consistent, not fleeting. Duckworth, Peterson, Matthews, and Kelly (2007) conceived the concept of *grit*, comprising passion and perseverance, to account for how goals can be pursued persistently over a long time.

Engagement with others leads to interpersonal relationships that can be satisfying and fulfilling. An engaged relationship is one in which people are present, participating, and interacting actively with one another.

Group Strengths (collective efficacy, social support). Group strengths include interpersonal relationships but are more extensive. For our analysis, these include all such activities in a group context, stopping short of the broadest level of involvement with major systems (which are considered in the following section).

By "group" I mean interactions occurring among several people who come together, interact, and coordinate their efforts for a shared purpose. Such arrangements include organizations and associations, support groups, task groups, training groups, planning councils, counseling and mental health groups, and so on. Using personal and interpersonal skills in group settings allows members to be productive participants and to benefit from their involvement. Collective efficacy and social support are key dimensions of group strengths.

Collective Efficacy. This is a group's shared belief in its conjoint capabilities to organize and execute the courses of action required to produce given levels of attainments (Bandura, 1997, p. 477). Collective efficacy emerges from self-efficacy, but it is not necessarily additive. A group needs to coordinate and integrate its resources properly, including the self-efficacy of individual members, in relation to presenting situations. That aside, and it is a large topic for research, collective efficacy is a group property. Beliefs about collective efficacy across group members can predict positive group performance (Little & Madigan, 1994).

Collective efficacy is found in many spheres of involvement. Political participation, social action programs, and social influence represent three such areas. Of particular value for prevention is assessing the capacity for collective efficacy in community-wide social change projects and in designing group enablement programs so that participants can exert their influence over community practices and positively affect the well-being of themselves and of the community.

Social Support. Social support exceeds the "support groups" element contained in Albee's original formula. By definition, support groups contain a small number of participants with a designated leader, and their purpose is to promote individual remediation and healing through intermember support. Millions of support groups and self-help groups (those meeting without a designated leader) exist in the United States, with the most famous being Alcoholics Anonymous. You can find listings of some of these groups in any community newspaper. By and large, that is a very good thing, indeed, as both support groups and self-help groups can be valuable for those involved.

Social support, however, is a broader concept than support groups. Although social support is a key mechanism in support groups—and all other kinds of groups—its significance is that social support is a general and critical process through which people connect and relate to each other in and out of organized group contexts. Social support can be thought of as a "psychological and emotional connective tissue" that serves to keep people in relationship, available to give and get help or simply to enjoy each other's company.

As I mentioned previously in relation to support groups, weak or absent social support sets the condition for negative conditions to occur. A recent study conducted by the Search Institute in Minneapolis of 6,300 seventh and eighth graders in Greater Cincinnati (Goodman, 2008) showed that only 20%–25% of the teens surveyed feel valued by adults. "Too many young people do not have adults in their lives in a sustainable relationship who stay by them through thick and thin over a period of years," said Shelby Andress, a senior consultant with the institute. Family support, community values, and adult role models are positive predictors of positive outcomes as they reinforce strengths through social support and encourage fewer risk-taking behaviors.

Higher rates of illness, accidents, and suicide are all associated with low social support. Lynch's work (1977, 2000) on the relationship between loneliness, a corollary of a thin social support system, and heart disease is informative and riveting.

System Strengths (ecological competence, advocacy). Humans lead their lives within systems. These human systems are organized settings and arrangements within which work and effort occurs. These systems may be tangible, brick-and-mortar structures (e.g., government office buildings), electronic (e.g., Web based), or may consist of a maze of related policies, procedures, and regulations (e.g., political or economic system).

Systems can be bewildering. I realize this abruptly whenever I need to locate the phone number of some governmental agency. Scouring the city phone book for the number can be like looking for a needle in a haystack. At such times I always wonder how a new immigrant must get along, a veritable "stranger in a strange land" (Heinlein, 1961).

Nonetheless, to get along in a complex society, a person needs to develop system skills. Accessing health care, paying taxes, locating the nearest express mail office, or reporting a work complaint—these and innumerable other system-oriented issues require knowledge, skills, and strategies. Moving beyond basic survival and subsistence skills demands more sophisticated approaches so that people can prosper within human systems.

Ecological Competence. Steele (1973) wrote about "environmental competence" in relation to people realizing their potential within physical settings. He maintained that too frequently people accept the status quo, tolerating inappropriate settings. By environmental competence, he was referring to a person's ability to (a) be aware of the physical environment and its impact, and (b) use or change the environment to better achieve goals, without harming others or the environment itself. Steele maintains that people have much more of a choice about their environment and how to use it than they realize (Conyne & Clack, 1981).

Ecological competence (Conyne & Cook, 2004) builds and broadens Steele's conception. It refers to a person's ability to function effectively within all the systems of life, from physical to procedural, to cultural, to electronic. Getting from point A to point E, being able to negotiate life's twists and turns, influencing improvements that would better the quality of life, and living life with economic efficiency—these all are examples of ecological competence.

Cultural competence (e.g., Leffert et al., 1998) is an internal developmental asset that can be thought of as a part of ecological competence. In our multicultural world and society, being able to function well with people who are diverse in settings that also are diverse is dependent on possessing and using cultural competence. For some experts, cultural competence is so central to counseling (and, by extension, other helping fields) that they term it a "mandate for the profession" (Arredondo, Tovar-Blank, & Parham, 2008) in the quest for the common good.

Cultural competence develops over time in individuals and organizations. It involves valuing diversity, being self-aware, and managing and prizing differences. For leaders of counseling and therapy groups, for instance, culturally competent leaders are aware of their own ethnic and cultural heritage, gender, socioeconomic status, sexual orientation, abilities, religion and spiritual beliefs, and values, and they respect differences (Association for Specialists in Group Work, 1998). To participate fully in our dynamic, diverse society, citizens from all walks of life need to develop sufficient competence in multicultural situations. Assessing their level of cultural competency, and ecological competency, in functioning within systems is important for prevention programming.

Advocacy. Systems are not always fair and equitable. Access to societal resources can be restricted. Barriers, such as racism, exist for many minorities and people who are poor.

Pitts (2008) urges that people don't need to "live with" an unjust justice system. He draws from an old Richard Pryor gag about a white couple seeing black people using drugs in a ghetto and saying "Tsk, tsk." Then they go home to find their son strung out on drugs. They cry, "Oh, my god, it's an epidemic."

These are differently held views, laden with bias and misperception. These inaccuracies arise from certain stated and institutionalized societal values, culture, policies, and structures, and their expression is experienced as being oppressive and exploitative by those on the receiving end. These behaviors harm human welfare, marginalize those affected, and limit their participation. As Vera et al. (2009) state:

> A person's race or ethnicity is not a risk factor in and of itself. Rather, the type of marginalization that a poor, Mexican immigrant child, for example, may experience within the school system contributes to a less than optimal learning environment, which may increase the temptation to leave school prematurely. (p. 109)

Advocacy is a social justice and social change approach used within a range of helping professions to promote needed system change and to support individuals. For example, the American Psychological Association's Guidelines on Multicultural Education, Training, Research, Practice, and Organizational Change for Psychologists (American Psychological Association, 2003) provide direction for how issues of culture and of oppressive systemic structures and processes can be included in the creation, application, and evaluation of prevention programs (D. W. Sue & Constantine, 2005). The American Counseling Association (2008a) details how advocacy can be delivered with and for clients, communities, and the public. These documents set directions for professional practice.

Advocacy also is a skill that citizens can use, or learn to use, to improve their lives and to prevent the continuation of unfair and inequitable policies and practices. They can attempt to effect change for themselves and others by identifying problems arising from a system (e.g., a local school's decision to excise extracurricular activities) and taking assertive action intended to reverse the action. Citizens can become informed about how to better manage their situation in relation to large systems, such as health care. For instance, Dr. Carolyn Clancy's column (Clancy, 2008) contains suggestions about health care, such as how men can become advocates in their own health care. Did you know, for instance, that for adult males in the United States: (a) one out of five have heart disease, (b) one out of three have high blood pressure, (c) three out of four are overweight, and (d) nine out of ten of lung cancer cases are due to cigarette smoking? The advocacy message is: "The single most important way you can take care of yourself and those you love is to actively take part in your health care. Educate yourself on health care and participate in decisions with your doctor" (Agency for Healthcare Research and Quality, 2008b).

Advocating for your strengths and those of others, without infringing on anyone's rights, is an important prevention strategy. For many, this approach seems unnatural, as counselors and other helpers typically are expected to be "nice" and not rock the boat. This inclination, termed the "nice counselor syndrome" (Bemak & Chi-Ying Chung, 2008), can work to vitiate efforts to advocate for strengths (as well as for social justice), thus cutting off one potential source of preventive influence.

Take a look at the following learning exercise related to advocacy.

LEARNING EXERCISE 4.4

Becoming a Strengths-Based Advocate

Increasing strengths is critically important in prevention. Program development personnel must learn to give specific attention to strengths because the tendency is to look for what is NOT working, what the deficits are. However, a strengths-based approach seeks to identify what is working well within a targeted population and then to figure out how to augment those assets.

Take a look at your own life, once again. It may be easier for you to identify what is not working so well; but this time, focus on what you do well, your strengths. How can you enhance them, use them for further improving your life, and become a strengths-based advocate for yourself and others?

Jot down your ideas below:

_____

_____

_____

Now that essential prevention concepts and criteria have been addressed, we move directly to consider program development and evaluation (PD&E). Section II, following, presents a collaborative, participative, culturally relevant approach.

Summary

This chapter concentrates on the original Albee incidence reduction formula and the adapted version. Incidence reduction is the gold standard for prevention programs due to the emphasis on stopping or reducing *new* problems and disorders. Prevention programs may be unable to accomplish that intention with regularity because of the challenges involved. However, I suggest that this is the place to aim while also making plans for other, more reachable goals, such as developing competencies and reducing deficits.

The adapted incidence reduction version expands and specifies the original formula. It provides program planners with focused direction for identifying problems to be prevented. The planning form that the adapted version has spawned is available in Appendix G. Further, its use is illustrated in Chapters 8 and 9.

Running through the previous four chapters on prevention have been many references to the importance of program development and evaluation in successful prevention interventions. The themes motivating this book are that (a) knowledge, skill, and experience in program development and evaluation are needed for conducting prevention programs successfully and (b) an incidence reduction, collaborative, participative, culturally relevant approach to program development and evaluation is best suited to prevention.

SECTION II

Program Development and Evaluation

*P*raxis is a Greek word referring to the reflexive relationship between theory and practice. Closer to home, the American philosopher and educator John Dewey emphasized the importance of learning and doing, where one without the other was but a partial approach. Undergirding the professional training in much of psychology is the model of the "scientist-practitioner," where knowledge without its practice—and the reciprocal informing of one by the other—is insufficient. So our philosophical and educational traditions point to the dynamic relationship between theoretical knowledge, on the one hand, and action on the other.

How does this brief foray into educational philosophy connect with our focus on prevention program development? Section I of this book centered on the theoretical and conceptual foundations of prevention itself. Although very important, knowledge about prevention by itself is inadequate preparation for being able to produce preventive interventions. Needed is a technology through which prevention knowledge can be channeled and applied, yielding a form of Theory + Action, if you will. This technology we will refer to as *program development and evaluation* (PD&E). Hence, we can describe this situation with another formula: Prevention Knowledge + PD&E Action = Preventive Interventions.

Section II contains two chapters that serve to define the underpinnings of a PD&E action technology. Chapter 5 explains some basic understandings about PD&E and the "AAEES" criteria of adequacy, appropriateness, effectiveness, efficiency, and side effects. Chapter 6 emphasizes the origins of PD&E in evaluation research and the evolving importance of framing PD&E within a community-based, collaborative, culturally relevant perspective.

Program Development and Evaluation

Basic Understandings

Chapter Overview

- Orienting to Program Development and Evaluation
- Defining PD&E
- Learning Exercise 5.1. Mix and Match
- Summary

Orienting to Program Development and Evaluation

The most frequently asked question I get about prevention goes something like this: "Okay, yes, I see that we should be doing more prevention. But how do we do it?"

After learning about what prevention is (Step 1—see the first four chapters), then moving to Step 2 becomes possible: learning how to do and evaluate prevention programs. This is where programming development and evaluation (PD&E) bursts forcefully through the door.

This chapter will begin by addressing PD&E somewhat generically, without giving particular attention to PD&E steps or to prevention. At this point we can be content with developing a basic understanding of the PD&E process. As the chapter proceeds, we will integrate important moderators of PD&E: concepts of community and cultural relevance. I contend that without these elements, PD&E is flawed. So, let's move ahead.

Defining PD&E

PD&E refers to "a dynamic method that harnesses and directs resources and forces toward desired and testable goal accomplishment." This definition, although succinct, needs some elaboration.

> *. . . Dynamic method.* The PD&E method consists of a systematic series of steps that are followed in order to produce a program or intervention that can reach established goals. This method is dynamic, subject to appropriate adaptation that is consistent with the ebb and flow that characterize any human system.

> *. . . Harnesses and directs resources and forces.* This dynamic method focuses on heightening forces that already may be present in a setting and/or on introducing innovation within the setting. In either case, the method needs to include processes of collaboration and participation, and be evidence based.

In the first case, taking advantage of naturally occurring forces, PD&E involves starting with natural settings, such as soup kitchens, YMCAs, nursing homes, schools, the natural resilience of a population, informal or indigenous sources of help in the community, and neighborhood parks and the everyday activities that take place in them. Programs are developed around ongoing activities that organically nurture, challenge, and support people in the setting, harnessing these salutary interactions to reach designated goals. By doing so, social competency is facilitated from existing dynamics (Gullotta & Bloom, 2003), rather than being introduced anew from the outside. This approach maximizes the important values of authenticity and participant involvement (Goldston et al., 2008).

The second case, where programs are created, is more frequent and typifies how PD&E generally is understood and practiced. Here, program developers move through a series of steps to institute a planned intervention within a setting in order to benefit participants. What is created needs to appropriately blend evidence-based, tested programs with local conditions and people. Special care needs to be taken in this type of PD&E process to involve setting participants throughout and to avoid what is an all-too-common tendency to insert and manage programs from the "top down," providing what planners think might be best based on research or on their own experience and expertise. Equal care needs to be given to program alterations that better fit community conditions while not stripping the tested program of its change-producing essence. This is a point we will return to later in this chapter and throughout the book.

> *. . . Toward desired and testable goal accomplishment.* Programs are intended to reach goals. They are the means to the end, whether they essentially facilitate existing forces or are formulated from evidence-based work. The program plan is constructed to allow for evaluation of goal accomplishment (outcome or summative evaluation) and of the fidelity of the program implementation process with the intended plan (process or formative evaluation).

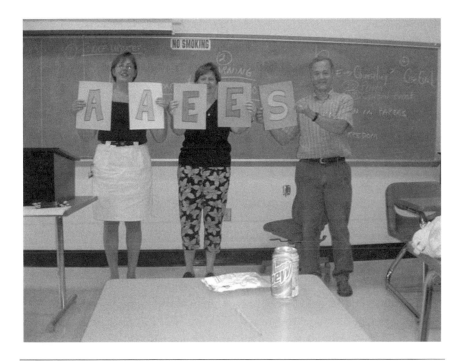

Figure 5.1   **A**ppropriateness, **A**dequacy, **E**ffectiveness, **E**fficiency, **S**ide Effects: Important Evaluation Criteria

Source: © John Conyne.

Whose goals and whose program are questions that are of fundamental importance. If PD&E processes are controlled and administered by external experts, then eventual success is compromised. Of deeper importance is that this top-down strategy renders useless the rich experience and skills of members for whom the program is intended. Such an approach is to be avoided in favor of one that embraces processes of collaboration, participation, and cultural relevance. This point, central to this book, will be elaborated once we move ahead.

Several evaluation criteria are important in these two types of evaluation. We consider these evaluation criteria next.

Yes, that's me in the photo above, with two student assistants (now graduates) in my course, Program Development and Evaluation. It's the last class session, and they have surprised me by bringing in the A-A-E-E-S signs. (I'll explain in just a moment.) They also had a song they had made up, which they passed out on a song sheet that everyone sang to the tune of "Old MacDonald Had a Farm." Here is an example stanza—you might try humming along with it:

> This class has been pretty cool. AAEES!
>
> Makes me want to work in school. AAEES!
>
> Is it adequate? Appropriate?
>
> Here effective, there efficient, everywhere a side effect.
>
> This class has been pretty cool. AAEES!

Now having at least read the lyrics above, you may have an idea of what the letters A-A-E-E-S stand for—that's right:

A: Adequacy

A: Appropriateness

E: Effectiveness

E: Efficiency

S: Side effects

A-A-E-E-S, then, are initials standing for program evaluation criteria (Craig, 1978), and they built the framework for the Program Development and Evaluation course I taught for decades—in which the song, mentioned above, appeared. Each criterion represents important questions to ask when determining if any program or intervention has been beneficial. The same criteria are among those that can be asked—and should be asked—not only at the end of a program but, also, at its beginning and all the way through its application. A-A-E-E-S are important criteria for program development and program implementation, too.

LEARNING EXERCISE 5.1

Mix and Match

Try matching the seven evaluative criteria with their brief descriptors now, before you read about them.

INSTRUCTIONS: Match criterion letters with the correct descriptor number and place in column 3:

Criteria	Brief descriptor	Correct match (letter-number)
(a) Context	(1) Last–fade	_____
(b) Adequacy	(2) Cost–value	_____
(c) Appropriateness	(3) Successful–unsuccessful	_____
(d) Effectiveness	(4) Right–wrong	_____
(e) Efficiency	(5) Oops	_____
(f) Side effects	(6) Strength–Weakness	_____
(g) Sustainability	(7) Surrounds	_____

In practice, these criteria are not mutually exclusive. They interact. A more accurate graphical depiction, then, would be: $A \times A \times E \times E \times S$. For instance, the bottom-line effectiveness of a program is dependent on its adequacy, appropriateness, and efficiency, and the side effects generated. However, for the sake of discussion, these criteria will be presented singly.

While being core considerations in PD&E, contemporary understanding suggests these five criteria may not tell the whole story. As research and practice have evolved, including considerations drawn from an ecological orientation (e.g., Bronfenbrenner, 1979; Conyne & Cook, 2004; Conyne, Crowell, & Newmeyer, 2008; Kelly & Hess, 1987), two additional criteria add substance: *Context* and *Sustainability.*

Let's take a closer look at these seven criteria for PD&E.

Context

Context is a "surrounds" criterion. It refers to the situation surrounding and influencing a population of interest. To some (e.g., E. Trickett, personal communication, January 2001), "context is everything." For instance, middle schools vary in relation to their contexts. One school located in rural, upstate New York is situated within a far different set of surrounding influences than another located in affluent Westchester County, just north of New York City. Same state, New York, but with dramatically different contexts. Variability occurs in relation to geography, of course, but also to climate, rural–urban environments, socioeconomic conditions, parental education, community values, job possibilities, availability of cultural and other opportunities, population density, racial and ethnic factors, and in many more ways. Going to school in one place or another, therefore, even at the same grade levels, can be quite different experiences due, to a large extent, to context.

The above discussion of contextual influences addressed proximal (nearby, close) ones, which tend to exert a continual press. Contextual influences also can be distal (far away), arising from national or international sources. As I write this section, economic conditions rank as the #1 concern among U.S. citizens in polls. Mortgage foreclosures, high gasoline prices, the unstable dollar (against the euro), and a volatile stock market all are combining to edge the economy toward recession. Many people are suffering or, at the least, having to cut back on spending and conserve. These macrolevel economic conditions add to the context of people's lives.

Therefore, it is important to assess proximal and distal contextual influences in relation to PD&E. All other evaluative criteria are moderated by their impact.

Adequacy

Adequacy is a strength–weakness criterion. A program or intervention needs to contain sufficient dosage and potency to produce the desired effect. Again, the Goldilocks Rule applies, so that neither too much nor too little of a program is needed, but it needs to be just about right. For instance, depending on its context (e.g., purpose, age of members) a 4-hour group counseling session may be too long, a 1-hour session too short, and a 2-hour session could be just about right. In another example, a program intended to improve reading levels that fails to include attention to social support among participants might be too weak. In prevention programs, achieving adequacy is dependent on involving people and settings with multiple components (methods, levels, sessions) that serve to interact and reinforce one another over time, such as those included in the Safe Schools/Healthy Students initiative (Elias, 1995) and in other evidence-based compendia. There must be "the right stuff" (Wolfe, 1979) to produce desired effects.

Appropriateness

Appropriateness is a right–wrong criterion. What makes a program successful for one population may not be suited for another one. Programs need to be culturally and ecologically relevant.

I told a tale (Conyne & Cook, 2004) that illustrates this concept. In the Copper Canyon region of the Mexican state of Chihuahua, some 7,000 feet above sea level, the native Tarahumara Indians are known for their running prowess. Up and down these deep canyons some of them run tirelessly and speedily, sometimes at marathon distances. The story goes that personnel of a major running shoe company thought they might capitalize on the running ability of the Tarahumara by letting certain prospects trade in their flat sandals for high-tech running shoes. Marketing opportunities loomed. After trying these new shoes out, however, they were returned by the Indian runners with the explanation that the shoes slowed them down. Besides, the runners said, they were much more comfortable in their customary ways.

Lesson learned. Cultural relevance is a key appropriateness concern. "Cultural invasion" needs to be avoided, where outside experts inflict their best intentions—even when evidence based—without the consent and participation of local people. Appropriateness of an intervention depends on matching it closely with characteristics of the population (and setting) for whom it is intended. Advancements in multicultural counseling and in diversity (e.g., APA, 2002; Association for Specialists in Group Work [ASGW], 1998; D. W. Sue, Arredondo, & McDavis, 1992), in best practice guidelines for prevention (Hage et al., 2007), and in culturally relevant prevention (Reese & Vera, 2007) have raised awareness about the need for exercising appropriateness in interventions and programs and have provided guidelines to improve that practice.

Considerations of appropriateness and of context, discussed above, are similar but with the following difference. Context refers to situations surrounding a population, whereas appropriateness refers to the population itself. What values do members hold? What cultural practices and beliefs tend to characterize population members? What language is spoken? What racial and ethnic characteristics describe the population? What traditions are in place? A substance abuse program that has been shown to be successful with a white, middle-class population would need to be altered (without losing its core elements) to more appropriately fit a Native American population, for instance. A culturally specific program, such as the "Fathers of Tradition" for Native American men (White Bison, 2007), might speak more directly to that population.

Effectiveness

Effectiveness is a successful–not successful criterion. In fact, there can be levels of success, too, so the question of effectiveness often is not strictly black or white in nature. A program can be somewhat successful, for instance, rather than judged as being totally unsuccessful. One way to judge if a program is effective is to determine whether most of its goals have been realized by participants.

As mentioned above, two types of program evaluation are conducted to determine success: (a) process or formative evaluation, which is concerned with how a program is being delivered in relation to its plan; and (b) outcome or summative evaluation, which is determined by evaluating program results in relation to program and individual goals that shaped the program's delivery.

As we have seen in earlier discussions of evidence-based programs, rigorous research and evaluation of program outcomes is considered the "gold standard." Thus, it is treated as a kind of "super criterion," in relation to the others. Efficiency, discussed next, easily wins the equivalent of the Olympic silver medal, because cost effectiveness is such a high priority.

However, the other criteria cannot be overlooked or minimized in their own importance; in fact, at times they may assume overriding significance. For instance, if a proposed program does not mesh with the values and traditions of participants, its inappropriateness is likely to yield program noncompliance or rejection and threaten program effectiveness. Remember the Tarahumara example of cultural invasion. In case that wasn't enough, here's another instance. In the Hawaii of the 1830s, missionaries convinced Queen Kaahumanu that the hula dance was "lewd" and immoral, resulting in it being banned for nearly 30 years (American Counseling Association, 2008b). Happily, hula dancing has been back in full force for 140 years or so, reaffirming an important cultural tradition and bringing untold enjoyment to many island visitors!

Reese (in Horne, 2008) pointed to an observation of Green (2007): "If we want more evidence-based practice we need more practice-based evidence." This is a call for participatory research and evaluation that is conceived and conducted within cultural and situational realities and where research and practice are mutually informed (Green & Ottoson, 2007). It also is an invitation for the evaluation of programs or policies through criteria developed in the field and for conducting research on how to influence provider organizations to implement programs that are empirically supported (Biglan, Mrazek, Carnine, & Flay, 2003).

Programs that are conducted to fit the context and match community and population characteristics need to be matched by research and evaluation that reflect those dimensions, as well. This is an important and recurring theme.

Kazdin (2008) recognizes the renewed emphasis within psychology and other disciplines to better link effective treatments with effective practice—not only to develop a stronger connection, but in order to enhance knowledge and improve care. Reese points out that science is much more than significance levels, effect sizes, and randomization. Although adherence to scientific methodologies is important, doing so sometimes is an aspirational quest, given real-world challenges (Conyne, 2004). Scientific methodologies need to be conducted, and perhaps modified, to fit the context and be responsive to changing conditions that are endemic to any community-based project (Vera, 2008; Vera et al., 2007).

Efficiency

Efficiency is a cost–value criterion. Following an expression of President Harry Truman, efficiency has been described as yielding "the biggest bang for the buck." A program can be effective but not efficient. How is that so? Imagine two autos, each of which runs well and are of similar size and weight. They can be driven between two points at the same rate of speed. However, one costs $40,000 and gets 18 miles to the gallon. The other costs $14,000 and gets 26 miles to the gallon. The first burns premium fuel, whereas the second uses regular (to make the example even more stark, imagine the second car as a hybrid or an electric car). Each automobile moves people to their destinations effectively, but efficiency clearly favors the second vehicle. The cars may not be equivalent in terms of attractiveness or perceived status, although these attributes can change over time, and they may or may not matter to the driver. In any case, in terms of efficiency, the greater bang for the buck goes to car #2.

Considerations of efficiency are always important with programs in mental health and education. We may all wish this situation were not so forcefully in place, although efficiency is an important criterion, nonetheless. It would be wonderful if funding support for our interventions were more generous. But that is not the case. Intended programs must be lean and parsimonious in terms of resources needed.

Indeed, efficiency is an especially important criterion in times of scarcity, where resources are few and competition for them is high. Budgets in health care and education always are restricted, but during economic downturns, they become particularly squeezed, in fact, often being among the first to be reduced. Grant funding sources look for proposals that show promise of effectiveness but also that are taut. Finding ways to "do more with less," a frequently expressed phrase today (some would lament, ad nauseam) demands close attention to questions of efficiency when designing and delivering quality programs. All things considered, efficiencies can be found when designing programs around activities and events endemic to a setting and by keeping imported resources to a minimum.

Side Effects

Side effects are an "oops" criterion. Program planners keep "main effects" in mind. What are the goals? How will we reach those goals? Were we successful in reaching those goals? However, as scientists and the public both have learned, occasionally with catastrophic impact (think of occasional air traffic control errors due to understaffed conditions), unintended effects always attend planned interventions.

Side effects in counseling are common. How clients respond and react to counseling interventions cannot always be predicted. A group member who learns in group how to become more assertive finds that his boss is not happy about this new behavior, and demotes him. Medication side effects can lead to troubling behavior that sometimes can become serious. Including mentoring in a prevention program sometimes results in the mentor gaining at least as much as and sometimes more than the mentee, a phenomenon known as the "helper-therapy principle" (Riessman, 1965).

Side effects occur in everyday life, too. One unintended effect that is very contemporaneous relates to the public's legitimate concern with "greening" the environment. Compact fluorescent lamps (CFLs) are able to save considerable money over time, compared to incandescent light bulbs, and they are beneficial to the environment because their usage generates smaller amounts of greenhouse gases. Many citizens have purchased these at initially higher costs (doing so will be mandated in 2016), being interested in cost savings over time and in environmental protection. However, there is no such thing as a free lunch, which is another way to think of side effects. Recently uncovered is the problem of how to dispose of these CFLs, because they contain small amounts of one of the deadliest elements, mercury. Special disposal is needed. In addition, if broken accidentally, a CFL releases the mercury, leading to a serious environmental hazard requiring special and costly cleanup.

Side effects also can be positive. I reported on ways that group leaders who make inevitable mistakes and errors, when engaging in deep processing, can learn from them to practice at higher performance levels (Conyne, 1999). Think of how Alexander Fleming discovered penicillin serendipitously from the mold encrusting a discarded petri dish. Or of Art Fry singing in the church choir, needing place markers for the upcoming hymns. He realized that the glue developed by his 3M colleague, Spence Silver—and thought to be a failure because it didn't stick very well—might be put to use to temporarily secure note reminders or place markers like he needed in the choir. After some experimentation, voilà—"Post-it notes" became ubiquitous.

In general, side effects are everywhere, too. The trick is to anticipate them better in planning programs. Every night during the televised evening news, a series of commercials for various pharmaceutical treatments inundates the hapless viewer. Because these also may appear at other times, if you watch any television at all you have been exposed to at least some of them. After touting the benefits of the medication being advertised, say it's to treat high cholesterol, then comes the long list of side effects. I'm making this up now in a burst of "truthiness" (i.e., intuitive, "gut-knowledge," not necessarily in keeping with any facts or logic, à la Stephen Colbert), but the list is probably not far off in accuracy: nausea, bloating, muscle pain, stiffness, dizziness, loss of consciousness, toe rot, bloody stools, horns—goodness, who knows what else? These are potential side effects of taking the main effect medicine, and sometimes they can be very rough, indeed.

In another case, many college campuses have announced themselves as being "dry" campuses, with penalties in place for alcohol violations. On the surface this community-level prevention policy and set of accompanying procedures may seem to be sensible and necessary as a way to lower the incidence of alcohol problems among students.

This is, of course, no small problem. Hingson, Heeren, Zakocs, Kopstein, and Wechsler (2002) report that 1,700 college students between the ages of 18 and 24 die each year from alcohol-related unintentional injuries and another 599,000 are injured inadvertently under the influence of alcohol. Equally alarming figures pertain to assault, sexual abuse, unsafe sex, academic problems, and health and mental health concerns.

But the problem is that there can be side effects of dry campus policy, or of any intervention. For fear of being "rung up," some students shy away from seeking help for another student who may have overdosed on alcohol or some other drug, choosing instead to let them (hopefully) recover without getting the emergency help they might need. This policy side effect is unintended and can be consequential. Recognizing the problem, some colleges have instituted an amnesty provision in their dry campus policy that would permit reporting emergency cases without penalty.

Unintended side effects can be reduced through vigilance during the planning process, by asking such questions as: What might happen that we haven't considered? What could go wrong that we haven't thought of yet? What might we be able to take advantage of, it if occurs?

Sustainability

Sustainability is a "last–fade" criterion. Program effects, when found, are subject to deterioration. They are difficult to maintain over a long stretch due to the tendency of an effect to wither without the continued program and in the face of changing personal and environmental conditions over time. Recognizing this propensity, program components need to be designed to promote the possibility that impacts will be maintained over time. As well, parallel evaluation procedures need to be sensitive to measuring postprogram effects. Booster sessions have been found to be useful in promoting sustainability, matched by accompanying evaluation points. Moreover, programs that have been created by or in collaboration with community members hold a greater likelihood of sustainability due to the direct stake of participants in the process and to their firsthand observation of positive changes (Goldston et al., 2008).

Summary

Program development and evaluation (PD&E) is a set of procedures for creating and evaluating any counseling intervention. It is not restricted to prevention, although the approach I will present later in this book is particular to prevention PD&E.

PD&E is essential to launching interventions that can make a difference in the lives of people and in society. Seven PD&E criteria were discussed in this chapter: (a) Context, (b) Adequacy, (c) Appropriateness, (d) Effectiveness, (e) Efficiency, (f) Side effects, and (g) Sustainability. These seven criteria provide a pragmatic framework to guide developing, conducting, and evaluating any intervention.

What gave rise to these criteria? How can they be implemented in practice? How are community-based and culturally relevant processes included? How is evidence-based practice included? These issues will be addressed next.

CHAPTER 6

Community-Based, Collaborative, Culturally Relevant PD&E

Chapter Overview

- Sources for PD&E
- The Role of Community, Collaboration, and Cultural Relevance in PD&E
- Learning Exercise 6.1. True–False
- Learning Exercise 6.2. Community Collaboration in Program Development
- Learning Exercise 6.3. Being Attuned to Cultural Relevance
- The Role of Evidence-Based Practice
- Learning Exercise 6.4. Evidence-Based Practice
- Summary

Sources for PD&E

PD&E emerges from the broad field of program evaluation, which contains a variety of theories and models that are supported by scholarly research and publications. The intent here is not to focus on the field of program evaluation but to draw from it generic applied PD&E steps that seem particularly useful, with some modification, in prevention. Certain program evaluation sources have played a larger role than others in informing this direction.

These sources, each to be briefly summarized in a moment, are (a) PRECEDE-PROCEED; (b) utilization-focused evaluation; (c) context-input-process-product;

(d) differential social program evaluation; (e) effectiveness-based program planning; (f) HIP Pocket Guide to Planning and Evaluation; (g) Collaborative for Academic, Social, and Emotional Learning implementation cycle; (h) student service program development; and (i) transformative research and evaluation.

PRECEDE-PROCEED model (Green & Kreuter, 1999). This model contains a comprehensive framework for assessing health and quality of life needs (PRECEDE) and for creating, delivering, and evaluating health promotion and other public health programs intended to meet those needs (PROCEED). This model's attention to ecological variables within an informed, cyclical approach provides strength.

Utilization-focused evaluation (Patton, 1997). This comprehensive approach is centered on the application of program evaluation findings by intended users, a focus that permeates it from beginning to end. The emphasis on involving stakeholder and primary users of program design and evaluation throughout the entire process of utilization-focused evaluation is an important contribution.

Context-input-process-product (CIPP) model (Stufflebeam, 2003). This comprehensive model considers formative and summative evaluation of programs according to four major elements: context, input, process, and product, with product organized by impact, effectiveness, sustainability, and transportability. The completeness and directionality (beginning with context through transportability) of a multistage CIPP evaluation is impressive, as is the incorporation of ecologically oriented concepts (context and sustainability).

Differential social program evaluation (Tripodi, Fellin, & Epstein, 1978). This framework indicates that social programs be evaluated by asking different questions timed to evolving program development stages (program initiation, program contact, and program implementation) and to distinct program evaluation stages (efforts, effectiveness, and efficiency). Specifying both program development and program evaluation stages along with sensitive questions timed for developmental progress in each stage provides for clarity and promotes effectiveness.

Effectiveness-based program planning (Kettner, Moroney, & Martin, 2008). This approach stresses the importance of monitoring in program planning, where programs are based on adequate and ongoing assessment. This commitment to effectiveness yields services to clients that are continually improved and provides a rich database for decision making.

HIP Pocket Guide to Planning and Evaluation (Craig, 1978). Specific program development and evaluation steps are defined that are based on usefulness and feasibility for application in daily circumstances. Six steps make up this approach: (1) Define the problem, (2) Set the objective, (3) Choose among alternative strategies, (4) Prepare for implementation, (5) Design the evaluation, and (6) Use evaluation information. The evaluation criteria A-A-E-E-S

(Adequacy–Appropriateness–Effectiveness–Efficiency–Side Effects), discussed earlier, were drawn from this source. The HIP model has been an important part of my teaching counseling graduate students program development and evaluation competencies for decades. The PD&E series of steps I reported (Conyne, 2004) is based largely on this approach.

Collaborative for Academic, Social, and Emotional Learning (CASEL) implementation cycle for socio-emotional learning (CASEL, 2003; Devaney, O'Brien, Resnik, Keister, & Weissberg, 2006). Ten steps are detailed for implementing socio-emotional learning (SEL) to transform leadership in a school (Elias, O'Brien, & Weissberg, 2006). These are: (1) Commit to school-wide SEL, (2) Engage stakeholders to form a steering committee, (3) Create and articulate a shared vision, (4) Conduct needs assessment, identify what already is working well, (5) Develop an action plan, (6) Select evidence-based programs and strategies, (7) Conduct initial staff development, (8) Provide socio-emotive skills instruction in classrooms, (9) Expand to whole school, and (10) Revisit and adjust. The overall set of steps and especially specification of commitment, engagement, visioning, and the incorporation of evidence-based approaches are welcomed contributions.

Student service program development model (Moore & Delworth, 1976). This tested model was part of the Western Interstate Commission for Higher Education initiative for improving mental health services on western campuses. The program development model contains five stages: (1) Getting the team formed and generating ideas using the Counseling Cube (Morrill, Oetting, & Hurst, 1974); (2) Core planning and development; (3) Pilot testing and deciding on offering; (4) Training and delivery procedures, program evaluation; and (5) Program maintenance and spinoffs.

Transformative research and evaluation (Mertens, 2008). In this approach, evaluation is conceptualized within a social justice framework. Research questions and issues are developed within the context of marginalized communities and by giving credence to community needs and evaluator-community partnerships.

The Role of Community, Collaboration, and Cultural Relevance in PD&E

PD&E, emerging from the discipline of program evaluation research, offers systematically organized methods for creating, delivering, managing, and evaluating interventions. However, success is not guaranteed. Too many initiatives based on PD&E methods have failed during development and are never brought to trial, are ineffective due to low participation and support, or when completed are not sustained or adopted elsewhere (Wandersman & Florin, 2003).

There are many reasons for these disappointments, but chief among them is the incapacity of PD&E approaches to genuinely include community members in collaborative processes throughout and to translate evidence-based approaches into culturally relevant forms. Therefore, PD&E can be improved by incorporating more fully attention to community and culturally relevant processes.

Attention to community, collaboration, and culturally relevant processes is not foreign to some existing approaches. For instance, see the steps for community health assessment in PRECEDE-PROCEED, attention to context and sustainability in CIPP, and engaging stakeholders in the CASEL implementation cycle. However, community involvement and cultural relevance are of such importance for enhancing readiness, involvement, satisfaction, adoption, success, and sustainability that they need to be centralized and prioritized within PD&E.

Traditional application of PD&E tends to be controlled exclusively by program personnel, with few exceptions. These exceptions need to become the norm. Collaborating with community participants meaningfully in all phases of PD&E promotes: (a) the identification of problems that have local value and import for daily living, (b) the reduction of programs that are perceived as being oppressive or exploitative by recipients, (c) the ability to better address social, health, and environmental inequities according to gender, race, ethnicity, and/or class that afflict many communities (L. Smith, 2005, 2008), and (d) the inclusion of those with the everyday, local expertise that is essential to accurately shape programs so they are culturally valid, useful, and sustainable (Jacobson & Rugeley, 2007).

The other side of the issue of assuring local community involvement in PD&E is that the efforts need to yield programs that are consistent with evidence-based research and are able to generate evidence-based findings. This demand is a complex one. To be locally and generally valid is not easily attainable, and often involves deciding on trade-offs along the way. Yet it is the aspiration.

LEARNING EXERCISE 6.1

True–False

1. Program development and evaluation emerges from the broad field of program evaluation.	T	F
2. Involving participants in all phases of program development and evaluation is a desired goal.	T	F
3. Utilization-focused evaluation emphasizes the usefulness of evaluation information that is produced.	T	F
4. Attention to community, collaboration, and cultural relevance are completely foreign to PD&E models.	T	F
5. Evidence-based PD&E is totally unrealistic.	T	F

Collaborating With Community Members

A *community* can be thought of as "a social group sharing common characteristics or interests and perceived or perceiving itself as distinct in some respect from the larger society within which it exists" (Flexner, 1993). Cincinnati, where I live, is made up of many distinct communities with probably the most well-known and historic being "Over-the-Rhine," the city's very first community, which is a contemporary flash point for crime and ground zero for gentrification. Our attention to community is as a locus for programming, for conducting PD&E, and from which participation in all phases of these two dimensions can come.

A community location can be compared with a laboratory, office, or other location of experts such as a university (unless the targeted community is the university itself). These "settings of the experts" are located away from the people and issues being studied or that are the intended recipients of the program.

Grounding activity within a community, while challenging due to changing conditions and weaker control, can unleash many other important positive forces. In fact, the power of community action cannot be disregarded. For an example, regardless of one's political leanings, consider the 2008 election to U.S. president of Senator Barack Obama: "Never underestimate the power of a community organizer and an organized community" (Baye, 2008, D-7).

Community location clearly and concretely communicates that the local community and its members are prioritized. It makes the program "real world," by definition. It allows for the possibility of community member involvement and participation. It opens opportunities for collaboration to occur among expert personnel and community members in the program. It fosters acceptance of and satisfaction with the program. It improves the likelihood of program success. It extends prospects for program continuation and sustainability of program effects.

Aspects of Community Collaboration

In Situ. Community-based programs increase the potential to improve local lives and settings when they are located in the community that is being addressed. Such a community location provides an ecological validity that cannot be matched otherwise. It opens the program to community resources and constraints directly and makes collaboration between program and community personnel a requirement. Although the real-world nature of a community location is invaluable because of its authenticity, it also brings unique challenges that need to be continually addressed, including readiness of the community members, fast-changing and unpredictable dynamics, and political pressures.

Locus of Control. What we are trying to do is to move away from PD&E that is essentially in the hands and control of program personnel separated from the community. This means strolling down from the "ivory tower" to the community and also climbing up from the community to the ivory tower. Both groups need to move. Initiation of this interchange can begin with either party, but openness to it is required by each.

Coequal Partnerships. Such mutual movement can lead to the desirable integration of science and experience that can characterize this form of PD&E, where scientists and community members become partners and colearners (Elden & Levin, 1991) and where "doing to" is replaced by "working with," as I mentioned earlier. This collaborative stance respects and benefits from the unique knowledge, skills, and experience from each side of the partnership. The theoretical knowledge and research abilities of the scientist can be joined with the practical, real-world local knowledge, skills, and experience of the community member. In such an arrangement it is inaccurate to restrict the term "expert" to program personnel alone. Expert contributions, of different types, come from each side to complement both. In fact, collaborative partners can be thought of as "coexperts."

Integration of Knowledge and Action. What Elden and Levin term "cogenerative learning" can emerge from program and community personnel collaborating, leading ideally to the cocreation of local and scientific information of value. Whether this ideal is reached is a function of many factors. Central among them is the initial mutual establishment of expectations that support the goal of producing information of value both locally and generally, and then developing and maintaining technical processes that contribute to its accomplishment.

Cyclical, Reciprocal Process. Working together effectively is based on developing and maintaining trust, a respectful partnership, and involvement throughout the PD&E process. In this approach, progress is continually reinforced by new data and experience while remaining true to core dimensions of the program.

PD&E often is thought of as a straight-ahead process. Step A leads to Step B to Step C, and so forth. Although this kind of linear thinking can be appropriate and helpful for teaching the major steps of PD&E, and we will take advantage of it for that purpose in this book, it is insufficient when applied in the complex and dynamic community. In practice, PD&E is not linear but cyclical, reiterative, and adaptive. The process can move back and forth, as conditions warrant, while moving generally forward as it follows a plan. Its steps serve as reference points to guide evolving adaptation as it is needed to meet changing circumstances. So, a planning council might define a problem to be addressed and feel comfortable with that definition. However, as planning members move ahead toward considering next steps, the information developed may sometimes cause them to redefine the problem. They then need to cycle back to do that before they can proceed. Or a set of goals identified may need to be modified because of budget cuts or staff changes or a community emergency of some kind. Program development and program evaluation are mutually influencing, not discrete and separate functions.

Strengths and Resources. Collaborating at the community level provides the means for more readily identifying and maximizing strengths and resources existing and available within the community and its residents. Working together provides an avenue for community members to express their capacities and translate their experience to inform program design and implementation in ways that scientific knowledge and expertise cannot. Community members can enhance their strengths and resources, becoming more empowered through their active engagement. As well, program personnel themselves can expand—or develop new—understanding and skills through their participation in the community. It is a win-win situation.

LEARNING EXERCISE 6.2

Community Collaboration in Program Development

1. Explain the benefits and the challenges involved in trying to obtain community involvement in prevention program development.

   Benefits: _____

   _____

   _____

   Challenges: _____

   _____

   _____

2. What abilities do you think would be helpful in promoting community collaboration? Where do you stack up in relation to them?

   Abilities: _____

   _____

   _____

   Self-assessment: _____

   _____

   _____

Aspects of Cultural Relevance

Genuinely conducted community collaboration yields cultural relevance, and vice versa. Developing positive working relationships between prevention program personnel and community members allows for the possibility of creating and implementing programs that are culturally valid and valued by the community. This point represents the nub of cultural relevance within prevention programs: *consistency between the programs themselves and how they were developed in relation to the beliefs, values, and preferred outcomes of community members* (Reese & Vera, 2007). Shaping prevention programs to attune them with cultural relevance is an important principle in the science and practice of prevention.

┌───┐

LEARNING EXERCISE 6.3

Being Attuned to Cultural Relevance

Reiss and Price (1996) observed that a prevention program must be reflective of and responsive to its community in order to be culturally valid. Vera et al. (2007) referred to this as an important litmus test, terming it the prevention program's "face validity."

What does it mean for a prevention program to be perceived by community members as possessing face validity? Give five examples of important characteristics that might generally need to be reflected in any prevention program to be culturally relevant.

Five characteristics of cultural relevance that I see:

1. _____

2. _____

3. _____

4. _____

5. _____

Now, discuss your list with another student. What do you find in common? Any differences?

└───┘

The Role of Evidence-Based Practice

Meaningful research results must be disseminated locally in ways that are understandable and can influence application potential. Ideally, research needs to be conducted also to allow significant findings to be disseminated more generally through established scientific and professional means (Israel, Schultz, Parker, & Becker, 1998). This commitment to dissemination in either case is too often given short shrift.

In terms of local application, often results are not translated meaningfully into terms and action steps that community members find understandable or useful. In terms of scientific spread, often results are produced that cannot meet the rigors of presentation and publication outlets. This "local-general" issue can be perplexing and needs to be kept in focus during PD&E.

Careful consideration of relationships between research and application is needed to produce research and programs that are both locally and generally important. In the following discussion of evidence-based practice, notice the attention given to cultural relevance.

Evidence-based practice (EBP), a term that spans efficacy and clinical utility, is central to a local-general connection. It combines the concepts of research efficacy and clinical utility.

Research efficacy refers to the strength of evidence indicating causal relationships between interventions and disorders. This is a scientific emphasis, with consequences for generalization.

Clinical utility draws from consensus about generalizing interventions with research evidence, their acceptability to clients, their feasibility, and their costs and benefits. This is a practice emphasis, with consequences for local application.

Evidence-based practice (EBP) combines these two sets of criteria of efficacy and utility. It is defined by the Institute of Medicine (2001, adapted from Sackett, Straus, Richardson, Rosenberg, & Haynes, 2000) as "the integration of best research evidence with clinical experience and patient values" (p. 147).

Evidence-based practice in psychology (EBPP) expanded the Institute of Medicine conception of EBP, giving fuller attention to client-related factors. The American Psychological Association Presidential Task Force on Evidence-Based Practice (2006) defines EBPP as "the integration of the best available research with clinical expertise in the context of patient characteristics, culture, and preferences" (p. 273).

Notice the contextual emphasis inherent in the APA definition of EBPP, with consideration given to the *characteristics, culture, and preferences of clients.* This connection is salient for PD&E approaches that are community based and culturally relevant.

Counseling, prevention, and other psychological services are most likely to be effective when they anticipate or respond to the recipient's unique "world." This world includes the client's

(a) specific problems;
(b) strengths and goals;
(c) chronological age and developmental history;
(d) preferences, beliefs, interests, values, and worldviews;
(e) characteristics, personality, gender, ethnicity, race, and social class; and
(f) the sociocultural and environmental context (APA Presidential Task Force on Evidence-Based Practice, 2006; Norcross, 2002; S. Sue, Zane, & Young, 1994).

These contextual influences are linked through the professional judgment of the practitioner with the best research available. Research findings considered are not restricted to any one model. Rather, this research can be produced through multiple methods, including: (a) efficacy, effectiveness, cost-benefit, epidemiological, and treatment utilization; (b) quantitative and qualitative designs, as well as clinical observation; (c) experimental and natural settings; and (d) process and outcomes studies. Systematic reviews, meta-analyses, effect sizes, and both statistical and clinical evidence are typically relied upon to identify the best available research (APA Presidential Task Force on Evidence-Based Practice, 2006).

A community-based, collaborative, and culturally relevant PD&E for prevention, the subject of this book, seeks to yield programs that are useful in the local community and that can be generalized to the scientific community, as well. Including EBP that is culturally relevant is a key aspect of such an approach.

The next learning exercise will assist you to think more closely about evidence-based practice.

LEARNING EXERCISE 6.4

Evidence-Based Practice

1. Evidence-based practice in psychology is defined as "the integration of the best available research with clinical expertise in the context of patient characteristics, culture, and preferences." How does this definition relate to research, on the one hand, and to context, on the other?

    _____

    _____

    _____

2. Circle below if the following statement is True or False: "If you are really serious about producing evidence-based prevention, then it is necessary to exclude cultural issues."

True	False

3. What is meant by the "unique world" of clients? What factors typically are included?

    _____

    _____

    _____

Summary

Program development and evaluation (PD&E) is a subset of evaluation research. In this chapter you read about different PD&E approaches that have emerged and that can be very helpful in practice. These include PRECEDE-PROCEED, *utilization-focused evaluation, CIPP, differential social program evaluation,* the *effectiveness-based* approach, the *HIP Pocket Guide,* the *CASEL* format, the *student service program development model,* and the *transformative research and evaluation* approach. In addition, the roles of community, collaboration, cultural relevance, and evidence-based practice were considered as they relate to PD&E approaches.

In the next chapter a prevention program development and evaluation (PPD&E) approach will be presented that seeks to integrate these various elements. A community-based, collaborative, and culturally relevant PD&E approach results that is particularly sensitive to prevention.

SECTION III

Ten-Step Prevention Program Development and Evaluation Approach

The four chapters of Section III are action oriented. They illustrate in concrete terms a 10-step approach to prevention program development and evaluation (PPD&E). In PPD&E, prevention and program development and evaluation are interconnected rather than being separate domains. Think of it this way: For effective preventive practice, PPD&E powers prevention along.

You will derive the most benefit from these upcoming chapters by defining and working with a prevention topic of your own. Even better, you can maximize learning by teaming up with others and together working on a prevention topic. You will encounter periodic process checks along the way that prompt you to examine your progress and that of your team—so having a team to work with will enable you to get the most out of this opportunity.

Chapter 7 shows how laying the groundwork for prevention occurs through eight planning steps that are loaded with process considerations. Beginning with establishing and maintaining a team (Step 1) through assessment (Step 8), the conditions for conducting prevention need to be nurtured, similar to how a gardener tills and nourishes her garden in preparation for growing flowers or vegetables. The clear focus throughout these eight steps is on process, highlighting the importance of community, collaboration, and cultural relevance in prevention program development and evaluation.

Chapter 8 moves to specific planning of how the prevention program itself can occur. Steps 9 and 10 of the prevention program development and evaluation approach are involved with specific planning of the prevention program itself, as well as how it will be evaluated. Step 9 is concerned with preparing and designing the prevention program, from generally defining problem identification (the adapted incidence reduction formula is introduced), setting the objective, choosing strategies, and detailing activities, tasks, responsibilities, and timelines. Note that Chapter 9 to follow returns to the step of problem identification to detail how examining incidence reduction in prevention can be done. Step 10 is concerned with designing the prevention program evaluation, with attention to assessing process and outcome and other elements. It centers on the question, "What resulted and how did it occur?" Creating a program evaluation plan provides the capacity to monitor the program (process or formative evaluation) to determine if program implementation is congruent with program intentions, and then to conclude if goals and objectives were met (outcome or summative evaluation). A particular concern with determining incidence reduction is to assess whether the prevention program contributed to a lessening in new cases of the problem that was addressed in the program.

Involvement in these steps can be rightfully thought of as the "nitty-gritty" of the prevention program development and evaluation process. All the i's get dotted and the t's get crossed as planning moves forward, circles back, and moves forward again. Planning needs to produce clear, concrete, and comprehensive outcomes, avoiding abstractions. As a 19th-century American Shaker might warn, this is *not* the time to be "superfluously fanciful" (Shaker Tour Guide, 2008). The photograph below illustrates the more desirable concept of parsimony, showing one way that the omnipresent Shaker wall pegs that routinely were featured in their buildings were put to use—hanging chairs, in this case upside down, and candles. Prevention program development and evaluation can well take a lesson.

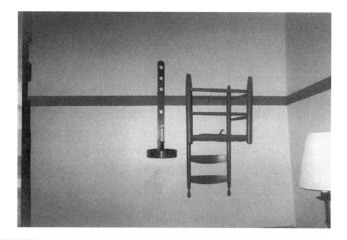

Figure III.1   Often simpler is better.

Source: © Robert Conyne.

The next chapter (Chapter 9) represents a "back to the future trip" by returning to the program design step of problem identification. Its contents detail how in prevention program development and evaluation the identified problem can be analyzed in terms of incidence reduction. This chapter is devoted entirely to applying the adapted incidence reduction formula to an example involving campus interpersonal violence.

Chapter 10 concludes the book by describing three programs in campus interpersonal violence prevention. Through interactive exercises, the chapter provides you with opportunities for applying your prevention program development and evaluation knowledge—and identifying your learning.

CHAPTER 7

Laying the Groundwork for Community, Collaboration, and Cultural Relevance Processes

Steps 1–8

Chapter Overview

- Getting Oriented to Prevention Program Development and Evaluation: The Three Cs
- Select Your Own Prevention Topic
- Learning Exercise 7.1. Working With Your Own Prevention Topic
- Steps 1–8: Laying the Groundwork for Prevention Planning—Developing Community, Collaboration, and Cultural Relevance
- Learning Exercise 7.2. Assessing Your Interpersonal Skills
- Learning Exercise 7.3. Conduct a Process Check
- Learning Exercise 7.4. Process Check #2
- Summary

Getting Oriented
to Prevention Program Development
and Evaluation: The Three Cs

We have been leading up to a PPD&E approach that embraces three processes, which we can refer to as the three Cs:

- Community based
- Collaborative
- Culturally relevant

The complete prevention PD&E approach is composed of 10 major steps that are divided into two groups: (a) Steps 1–8, which *lay the groundwork* for the focused prevention planning, and (b) Steps 9–10, where the *prevention program and its evaluation* are designed. Table 7.1 contains Steps 1–10.

Steps 1–8 should be completed before moving to the last two steps. Within Steps 1–8, however, the progression need not be absolutely sequential. It is presented that way simply for clarity of discussion. For instance, the approach could be started with Step 4 (explore related literature) and then move back to Step 1.

Table 7.1 Ten-Step PPD&E Model

A. LAY THE GROUNDWORK (Steps 1–8) for Community, Collaboration, and Cultural Relevance
STEP 1: Establish and maintain a team
STEP 2: Identify a potential community issue
STEP 3: Explore related professional literature
STEP 4: Develop a germinal, motivating idea
STEP 5: Engage stakeholder planning council
STEP 6: Create a shared vision and mission
STEP 7: Stimulate community readiness

STEP 8: Assess
    a. Conduct a local ecological assessment
    b. Search for evidence-based programs

B. IMPLEMENT AND EVALUATE (Steps 9–10)
STEP 9: Design the prevention program plan
STEP 10: Design the prevention program evaluation plan

Table 7.2   Lay the Groundwork (Steps 1–8) for Community, Collaboration, and Cultural Relevance

---

STEP 1: Establish and maintain a team

STEP 2: Identify a potential community issue

STEP 3: Explore related professional literature

STEP 4: Develop a germinal, motivating idea

STEP 5: Engage stakeholder planning council

STEP 6: Create a shared vision and mission

STEP 7: Stimulate community readiness

STEP 8: Assess
    a. Conduct local ecological assessment
    b. Search for evidence-based programs

This chapter will be reserved for these first eight preliminary steps. Table 7.2 contains only these first eight steps.

Applying the first eight steps lays the groundwork for specific prevention planning by emphasizing the processes of community, collaboration, and cultural relevance. Attend to how these three processes run through Steps 1–8 as you read the rest of this chapter. Implementing these steps lays the groundwork for prevention program development and evaluation in general and for an evidence-based approach to it that will be discussed in subsequent chapters.

Select Your Own Prevention Topic

As I have pointed out twice earlier (because it is so important), you will be able to enhance your learning about how to develop and evaluate prevention programs by first selecting a prevention topic you care about. Having done that, then you will be able to apply the procedures that will be presented to your own situation.

A step up from a personal exploration such as that described above is to join with others to form a team. Doing so will model the approach that will be presented, which leans heavily on collaborative team work. I strongly encourage you to implement one of these two approaches, with the second one preferred. The next learning exercise will assist you.

> ┌─ **LEARNING EXERCISE 7.1** ─────────────────────────────
>
> ### Working With Your Own Prevention Topic
>
> This chapter will lead you through a sequential series of prevention program development and evaluation steps (as you already know, though, in practice these steps may not occur in a strictly linear manner).
>
> You will get the most from this chapter by taking a moment now to select a potential prevention topic—say, preventing bullying in a seventh-grade class or preventing depression in recently unemployed workers—or, best of all, choose something that you care about very much.
>
> Then, work actively with your chosen prevention topic as you read each step. Imagine applying it to your situation.
>
> EVEN BETTER—If you can, get together with a few others who are reading this book to form a team and move through the steps together!

Steps 1–8: Laying the Groundwork for Prevention Planning—Developing Community, Collaboration, and Cultural Relevance

Step 1: Establish and Maintain a Team

(Reminder to readers: Here is where your team, addressed in Learning Exercise 7.1, will begin to be helpful to you as you move ahead.)

Developing a program requires many resources, including a base of support or a team. "Lone rangers" are usually unsuccessful in prevention. Indeed, acting as a solo agent virtually guarantees failure. The tasks are too complex. They demand experience and expertise that no one person possesses. In addition, sanction and resource support are essential for progressing. A team whose members learn how to function collaboratively can help develop and guide initiatives and obtain necessary support.

Interpersonal Skills. Accomplishing this step successfully takes skill and continual attention. Actually, the process begins with self-assessment of your attitude and skills. To form a base of support, or a team, requires interest and skills in working with others. In fact, the entire prevention planning process depends strongly on possessing a positive interpersonal attitude and skills. Great ideas need to be complemented by equally great attitude and skills. The crux of the matter for putting a team together is that interpersonal sensitivity and ability are forces that drive accomplishment, along with commitment to the prevention process. The initial question, then, is: "How interpersonally adept are you?"

Try your hand at the next learning exercise.

LEARNING EXERCISE 7.2

Assessing Your Interpersonal Skills

This learning exercise provides you with an opportunity to self-assess your existing interpersonal skills.

First, respond to the five questions below. Circle the number that best captures your general assessment, where: "1" = Never and "5" = Always, and then briefly explain:					
1. I enjoy being with other people.	1	2	3	4	5
2. I am effective when working with others on tasks.	1	2	3	4	5
3. Others tend to like spending time with me.	1	2	3	4	5
4. I like working with people in groups.	1	2	3	4	5
5. My skills are sufficient for working with others.	1	2	3	4	5

In Questions 6 and 7, jot down your thoughts:

6. In completing this exercise, I learned my interpersonal strengths seem to be:

_____

_____

_____

7. In completing this exercise, I learned I might need to improve the following:

_____

_____

_____

Sanction. At an early point it is necessary to obtain support for forming and maintaining a prevention team. Being a staff member of a mental health or educational agency affords a natural opportunity to acquire the legitimacy that is required. Of course, if one already occupies a staff role connected with prevention (e.g., coordinator of prevention services), the legitimacy usually is conveyed. Otherwise, it has to be created from within. In such cases, interpersonal skills need to be enhanced with organizational skills to advocate persuasively for formation of a prevention team.

Team Development. Once a team is formed, it is necessary to develop it. What makes a set of people a team is that they come to develop a sense of mutuality and interdependence. They join in a common purpose that defines their existence as a team, and they begin to accept that they are all part of the unit where each one is an important and meaningful contributor. The sense of cohesion that emerges in a well-functioning team is essential for maintaining the team over the long haul and for stimulating productivity (Fujishin, 2001).

Team Maintenance. After the team is developed, it needs to be maintained and sustained. This requires the team leader and its members to attend to the quality of team functioning (process) and to its success (outcome). Periodic review of how the team is doing can be very helpful for keeping progress on track. Assessments such as the following can be performed, using a 1–5 scale, where "1" = Never and "5" = Always:

A. *Team Members:*					
1. Show each other respect	1	2	3	4	5
2. Listen to each other	1	2	3	4	5
3. Show a positive attitude	1	2	3	4	5
4. Participate actively	1	2	3	4	5
5. Follow through on responsibilities	1	2	3	4	5
6. Help one another	1	2	3	4	5
7. Behave professionally	1	2	3	4	5
8. Deal well with conflict	1	2	3	4	5
9. Contribute ideas	1	2	3	4	5
10. Are helpful	1	2	3	4	5
B. *The Team:*					
1. Works well together	1	2	3	4	5
2. Accomplishes much	1	2	3	4	5
3. Stays on course	1	2	3	4	5
4. Does not waste time	1	2	3	4	5
5. Use its resources well	1	2	3	4	5

Assessments such as those above, which I just concocted but that are based on experience, are available on the Internet (e.g., CFED/REAL, 1993) and in professional sources (e.g., Kormanski, 1999). The keys are to develop a culture where team members are interested in considering and responding to these kinds of questions and will be likely to follow up on the feedback that emerges when they examine them.

Feedback that results from discussion of items such as these is used to identify next steps. These include: (a) what is working and should be continued and (b) what is not working so well and should be improved.

Later in this chapter you will find learning exercises that ask you to provide a "process check" of your work as a team. These are intended to assist you in keeping on track through short feedback sessions. Committing to such monitoring of performance can greatly assist a team and its members to function at its highest levels, perhaps even approaching the feathery notion that "teamwork makes the dream work" (Maxwell, 2002). Perhaps more realistically, performance monitoring can help avoid, or lessen, the many problems that can occur.

Figure 7.1 illustrates a case where a process check could be helpful. The team leader, shown at the end with the beard and glasses, just doesn't seem to "get it."

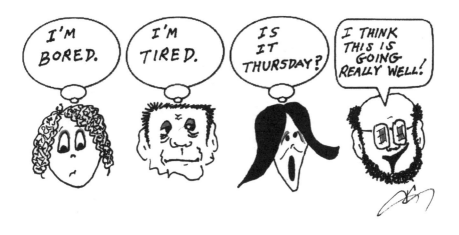

Figure 7.1   Adventures in Teamwork

Source: © John Conyne.

Team Facilitation. Of course, it takes good team facilitation to produce a well-functioning team that moves forward positively over time. This means someone who is competent in group process and group leadership. Too frequently leaders of task groups, teams, and committees are untrained in group work and have little or no supervised experience. It is no surprise, then, that their teams may not fare well. Training and supervised experience in group work helps a team leader to be able to think and behave in relation to the team as a whole, its intermember relationships, and with respect to individual members as the team seeks to meet its tasks and responsibilities (Conyne, 1989; Conyne, Crowell, & Newmeyer, 2008; Conyne, Rapin, & Rand, 1997; Hulse-Killacky, Killacky, & Donigian, 2001; Schwarz, 2002). Team facilitators need to be able to balance content and process dimensions that are sensitive to its various developmental stages. Hulse-Killacky et al. (2001) identified these task group stages quite simply as warm-up, action, and closure. As well, facilitators need to help the team to function well within the demands and resources of its external environment, allowing problem-solving and group processes to be mobilized, yielding prevention programs that work (Conyne et al., 1997).

Step 2. Identify a Potential Community Issue

(*Note to readers: Here is where you can select your own prevention topic to work on.*)

Community focus is "best." Prevention programs are intended to reach large numbers of people who are currently unaffected by a disorder. An example is preventing young teens who currently do not smoke or are not regular smokers from becoming addicted to cigarette smoking. The best place to reach these individuals is in and through their communities.

This strategy is "best" for a few reasons. First, it is parsimonious and cost effective to integrate programs within existing community structures and processes rather than to uproot people to participate in a program elsewhere. Second, taking advantage of naturally occurring processes and resources is authentic and genuine, not fabricated from the outside. Third, feasibility is enhanced when prevention practitioners work from within rather than from the outside or from the top down. The diminution of hierarchy results in a flattening out of typical power differentials and increases opportunities for shared activity.

All things considered, it usually is preferable to hitch a ride on naturally occurring community processes than to concoct new ones, however majestic they might be. The community strategy, then, is not to take people from their communities to participate in prevention programs but to introduce the prevention program within the communities themselves.

Becoming "Community Oriented": The Case of the Hammer. There are many communities, as was mentioned earlier. Neighborhoods, schools, work, religious settings, community organizations, and families all are among those that qualify. In addition, due to the Internet and its features such as e-mail, community forums, e-learning modes, blogs, and social networking channels, the definition of community needs also to include online options (in fact, for many today the sense of community may be experienced more often online than face to face). Therefore, however the concept of community is defined and realized, the team needs to become "community oriented" in its work.

This orientation can be challenging. Team members may have their own areas of expertise, their own successes with certain prevention programs and approaches. For instance, one member might have developed skills in working with problem-solving programs, another with bully busting, a third with substance abuse prevention.

Perhaps you know the story (told by Abraham Maslow) of the kid who discovered the hammer, a tool made for pounding and removing nails. He found the hammer so successful with nails that he thought it could be useful in all other projects, too. Hammering wood, though, did not work, and it didn't fare so well with screws, either. The moral of this tale is that a tool has specific uses and cannot be generalized. The kid learned by trial and error. Members of a prevention team need to keep that story in mind, too. Be guided by the community for what is needed, not by the tool that you may know so well.

Which local communities are experiencing problems? Or to ask it another way, what people are experiencing problems in their communities? This ecological question can be expressed as "People × Community." For convenience, we will refer to it as a "community issue."

Methods. The team needs to identify a community issue to explore that is important and might present a feasible preventive programming opportunity. In fact, the team might generate a number of potential items to explore at this point, eventually winnowing down to one or two to take forward more seriously.

This step can be conducted informally or formally. It involves scanning the community to identify an issue that is important and that would seem to hold the potential for developing a local program that could make a positive difference and that could be generalized.

Informal methods of identifying a community issue might begin with team members individually reporting their awareness of possibilities, drawn either from their own experience (e.g., "at my son's elementary school girls are finding it difficult to speak . . ."), through current case loads (e.g., "one of my clients reports many students use drugs . . ."), or through the media (e.g., "the paper this morning reported on high stress resulting from unemployment . . ."). Team discussions of this information may lead to crystallizing an issue to be explored further.

Formal methods of identifying a community issue involve conducting assessments. These might include individual interviews, focus group interviews, or survey questionnaires administered via paper and pencil or electronically. In all cases, those assessed should be knowledgeable about the issue being explored.

The point is not to conduct a thorough assessment—that comes later (see Step 8). Rather, the purpose now is to gather and consider fairly easily obtained information about community issues that seem to reflect real situations. Examples include childhood obesity, failing schools, high rates of suicide or violence, community fragmentation, and elder abuse. There are so many possibilities.

Step 3. Explore Related Professional Literature

Let's say Step 2 led your team to identify high rates of local community violence as a possible focus. What is the related professional literature on this topic? What studies have been reported? Are there hypotheses or even theories about community violence? Have causal or contributing factors been identified? What populations seem most at risk locally, nationally, globally? Are there different types of community violence? Is any of it preventable? Are there any preventive approaches that have been shown to work? How have these been developed? What results have been shown?

It is helpful when tackling complex tasks, such as a professional literature review, for team members to agree to handle certain tasks. For instance, one person might explore the Internet, another the local university library. Or if subtopics have been identified already, they could be assigned to different team members: relational violence, cyber-violence, bullying, racial violence, suicides, and so on—whatever might have been identified in the community assessment.

Of course, there is no such thing as a "free lunch." If assignments are differentiated, then what is produced needs to be coordinated. Indeed, coordinating and integrating team member functioning is a general and ongoing challenge. In the case of a differentiated literature review, obtaining and pulling together information into a usable and meaningful product can be taxing—or rewarding, depending on how it goes. If you've ever worked on a team-based project, you can relate to this matter. It is helpful to have a system to follow.

Problem-based learning (PBL) suggests such a system for team-based work (Duch, Groh, & Allen, 2001; Savery, 2006) It involves members asking questions, such as:

- What do we know already?

- What do we need to know?

- How can we access it?

- Who will do what?

- By when?

- How will the information be shared?

- Who will organize it?

- When will it be presented for consideration?

The information acquisition and compilation process can be aided or harmed by using an electronic learning resource, such a Blackboard (Bb; http://www.blackboard .com/us/index.bbbn) or WebCT (http://www.webct.com/webct). Those with access to these kinds of e-learning systems enjoy the capacity to communicate their research and interact between scheduled team meetings. This advantage can accelerate the search process and the coordination of material that is generated. However, users need to agree and comply with patterns for using these systems. If one person fails to keep current, however that may be defined, then a breakdown will occur. As well, users need to be cognizant of communicating with each other clearly and positively, not falling prey to blasting off emotionally when frustrated (I have seen this happen, and it can produce lasting scars).

At any rate, exploring professional literature—getting, coordinating, and discussing it—provides an additional helpful level to the program development process.

Step 4. Develop a Germinal, Motivating Idea

The PD&E process could well begin at Step 4, and then move "backwards" through preceding steps. Or the process might move to this step from earlier ones. The sequence is a matter of circumstance, and it is cyclical.

For the moment, we will work with an example based on a university campus context. Suppose you are a counselor in the university counseling center with the role of outreach coordinator. In this role you are responsible for coordinating the efforts of other staff to develop, deliver, and evaluate programs that are intended to prevent student psychological and educational problems while promoting growth and development.

Let's assume Steps 1–3 have been accounted for in planning. A brief summary follows:

Example Step 1: Team formation. You have established an outreach team in the counseling center consisting of five professional staff and two interns, each devoting 25% of their overall effort to this function. The team has developed its internal strength to move to next steps.

Example Step 2: Identify a potential community issue. Through informal assessment and discussion of local events and situations, your team has identified prevention of relationship violence as a potential issue to address. Data from counseling caseloads, reports in the school newspaper, and data from the campus Sexual Response Assault Team all indicate that relationship violence is an issue of high concern on campus.

Example Step 3: Explore related professional literature. The team has explored some of the professional literature related to this topic. Numerous sources were identified, read, and discussed dealing with relationship violence, including the document *Campus Sexual Assault: How America's Institutions of Higher Education Respond* (Karjane, Fisher, & Cullen, 2002). Various forms of relationship violence were noted, including occurrences during dating and courtship, alcohol-induced aggression, rape and sexual assault, oppression of gays and members of minority groups, roommate conflict, student–faculty relationship conflicts, suicide and homicide, and daily microaggressions.

By now the outreach team is arriving at some certainty that the general issue of preventing relationship violence on campus is worthy of pursuit, as it is supported by both local and national sources. The task now is to collaboratively produce a "germinal idea," that is, one that can serve to stimulate and frame next steps.

This need can be accomplished in three ways, through (a) informal discussion, where information and ideas are shared and analyzed, leading to the idea; (b) applying idea-creating devices, such as brainstorming or force-field analysis, that can serve to stimulate and organize the information that is generated; and (c) using both approaches. Whichever way is selected, the process of developing germinal ideas can be involving and lots of fun. Team members usually enjoy this PD&E step.

I want to introduce you to an idea-creating device that was mentioned in the preceding chapter and is sensitive to prevention: *Dimensions of Counselor Functioning Cube* (Moore & Delworth, 1976; Morrill, Oetting, & Hurst, 1974). This device is especially helpful when spinning out initial thoughts and developing possibilities. It serves as a kind of structured brainstorming approach. At the same time, using the Cube may not fit all situations. Treat it as an elective option, its use dependent on local conditions.

In my view, publication of the Cube (Morrill et al., 1974) represented a milestone in understanding the possibilities for counselor functioning. Why? It exploded the prevailing conception of what a counselor could do, including not only the familiar mode of individual, remedial, direct counseling but also lesser known ways, such as community, prevention, and consultation applications. In fact, the Cube projected 36 different counselor functions as being possible and desirable, not just the "one-main-one" in which one counselor worked with one client who presented a psychological or educational concern—or what I have termed the "counseling services paradigm" (Conyne, 2004).

The Cube is organized by three dimensions for counselor intervention: (a) intervention *purpose* (remedial, preventive, developmental), (b) intervention *method* (direct, consultation and training/indirect, media), and (c) intervention *target* (individual, primary group, associational group, community/institution).

Brief Definitions of Cube Dimensions Applied to the College Campus

Purpose of Intervention. Counselor interventions are conducted to correct existing psychological or educational deficits (*remediation*), to avert the emergence of new cases of deficits (*prevention*), or to build strengths to ward off deficits and contribute to a happier and more positive life (*development*). Note that the development purpose can be viewed as a way to reach prevention goals.

Method of Intervention. Counselor interventions can be delivered to targets (or recipients of service) by professional staff (*direct*); through others such as paraprofessionals, peers, or volunteers (*consultation and training [C&T], alternatively termed "indirect"* method); or through technology, whether print or the various electronic forms such as CDs, e-learning, the Internet, or television (*media*).

Target of Intervention. Counselor interventions can be aimed at one person's thoughts, feelings, or behaviors (*individual*); at close, ongoing, face-to-face groups such as roommates, couples, and families (*primary group*); at groups formed for specific task purposes, such as clubs, Greek organizations, residence halls, classrooms, and academic departments (*associational group*); and at the entire campus (*community or institution*).

Of particular interest for us are the *prevention and development purposes* of intervention and how they may interact with varying levels of intervention target and intervention method. In our example of relationship violence, prevention programs would seek to forestall the emergence of new cases or reduce the rate at which they occur.

Using the Cube Model for Developing a Germinal Idea

Brainstorm Purpose of Intervention by Target of Intervention. To use the Cube model, bring the planning team together to cast the information it has developed within the framework of the Cube. As well, the model can be used to generate new ideas. Conyne (2004) suggests as a first step that the team concentrate on prevention and development purposes across all levels of target.

Cells are designated by abbreviations (e.g., Cell P–AG = **Prevention–Associational Group**):

	Purpose of Intervention	
	Prevention (P)	*Development (D)*
Target of Intervention		
Individual (I)	___P–I_____	____D–I_____
Primary group (PG)	___P–P_____	____D–P_____
Associational group (AG)	___P–AG_____	**___D–AG_____**
Community (C)	**___P–C_____**	___D–C_____

The goal at this point is to generate many potential interventions. The accent is on production of possibilities. These then will be refined for quality using the evaluation criteria discussed earlier of context, adequacy, appropriateness, effectiveness, efficiency, side effects, and sustainability. Referring to our case of relationship violence at a university, let's imagine two examples that emerge from this process. They are highlighted above and abbreviated as P–C and D–AG.

For a P–C intervention (prevention purpose targeted at the community), our fantasy team came up with this possible intervention: "Lower the incidence of sexual assault by developing a positive campus culture focused on healthy relationships" (note it does not indicate the method to be used).

For a D–AG intervention (development purpose targeted at an association group), the team thought of this possible intervention: "Bolster fraternity and sorority members' capacity to relate positively with each other by improving their communication skills" (note it does not indicate the method to be used).

Brainstorm Method of Intervention. After generating possibilities for intervention based on interactions of Purpose and Target, consider the method of delivery for each one.

Method of delivery for purpose and target interventions:

Direct method _____

C&T/Indirect method _____

Media method _____

The question here is how might prevention and development programs be delivered? Returning to our examples, our team might come up with the possibilities highlighted:

P–C intervention:

Purpose: Lower the incidence of sexual assault

Target: Campus community

Method: Media campaign

D–AG intervention:

Purpose: Improve relational skills

Target: Fraternity and sorority members

Method: Conduct problem-solving communication skills workshops using psychoeducational group processes

What is produced through this process, while still tentative, should provide enough direction to allow for movement through the ensuing steps.

LEARNING EXERCISE 7.3

Process Check #1

It is important to pause periodically to consider how you and your team are functioning together as you work on the task at hand. Ask these questions:

- How are we doing?
- What's working?
- What's not working?
- How can we continue to improve our functioning?

Step 5. Engage Stakeholder Planning Council

Now the team has something to share with others in the community that they might find at the very least interesting and even compelling. The goal is to broaden beyond the team to establish a representative collaborative of community stakeholders who can plan a prevention program to address a significant local issue. The term *community stakeholders* refers to people who influence and are influenced by the community. Stakeholders often hold positions of importance or they have earned credibility through some other form of contribution. This group of people will become the core planning and coordinating council for the entire project.

Take time with this step, sometimes a few months. Jacobson and Rugeley (2007) report on how the *Finding Solutions to Food Insecurity (FSFI)* project took 4 months to establish a steering committee, involving recruitment and other forms of preparation. Members should be carefully selected, and effort needs to be devoted to helping them to form a working team (Schwarz, 2002). Members of this team (or planning council) most likely will come from various sectors of the community and from professional disciplines. The key is to bring together people to work together who (a) care about the issue, (b) represent constituencies involved with it in some meaningful way either practically or academically, (c) are interested in working collaboratively, and (d) can commit to the process over time and are supported in their commitment.

At first there might be barriers to participation that will need to be addressed. Because potential members come from different levels and places, they often bring with them some discrepant views and ways of doing things. It will be necessary to address issues of power, status, and difference in moving ahead, as well as to remove other roadblocks to participation. Something on the surface as simple as where meetings will be held may be reflective of cultural and status differences.

Creating and nurturing a working environment of mutual support and respect for diversity are important for a successful planning group. Helping everyone to gain appreciation for the value of each other's ideas and contributions is needed, where the concept of co-equal participation eventually becomes a mind-set. This will help develop an "inclusive space for teaching-learning" (Jacobson & Rugeley, 2007, p. 28), a perspective that supplants a one-way control of information with dialogue, collaboration, and mutuality (Finn & Jacobson, 2003). Such an inclusive space allows for both scientific information to be shared as well as knowledge drawn from people's lived experience. Both are useful for program development.

Step 6: Create a Shared Vision and Mission

Council members need to collaborate on producing both a vision and a mission. Doing so will help motivate them and keep them on track, as well as provide a concrete means for communicating their efforts to the broader community.

Vision. Abraham Maslow, the progenitor of humanistic psychology, noted that "the basic question is what vision do you aspire to?" (in Collins & Porras, 1997, p. 234). The planning council needs to answer that question, also. It is related to, but different from, *mission*, which is concerned with the question of why the group exists. A *vision* is a "mental picture of the future that a group seeks to create" (Schwarz, 2002, p. 27). It is the view of what's possible (Ballard, 2008). Thus, a vision needs to be inspirational, capable of evoking a clear image that is easily recalled and can be readily communicated to others. This vision needs to be engaging, serving to motivate people to work over the long haul. It needs to be created, for sure, but it also needs to be continually articulated to planning council members and to those outside it.

Mission. A planning council can define its mission by answering the question: "Why do we exist?" This is an important question, one that many groups and teams never quite get to consider.

A mission statement serves both internal and external purposes. Internally, it serves as an anchor point that provides sustained intentionality and direction over time. It is meant to direct the development of goals, strategies, and tasks. It allows for determining if the group is staying on course and if it was successful in the end. Externally, the mission statement can be used to communicate beyond the planning council to others who may be interested, to those whom planners aim to influence, and to provide legitimacy to a project, and a mission statement can assist in acquiring resources (Ballard, 2008).

A mission statement can be drafted in a variety of ways, but it should avoid being either too vague or overly specific. A statement of "We aim to improve human relationships" lacks sufficient specification for a mission statement, but might be suitable for an inspirational vision statement. A mission is more operational and might be: "Our agency will collaborate with others in the community to reduce interpersonal violence through preventive services." Here, you see a bit more definition without including detailed applications.

Some other types of mission statements, however, include concrete strategies for accomplishing the mission. In an example drawn from Ballard (2008), a university (SU) counseling center's mission was "to provide a wide range of services free-of-charge to SU students . . . including *screening and assessment, outpatient therapy for individuals and couples, crisis intervention* [italics added] . . . while seeking to foster a campus environment that promotes healthy behaviors and outstanding academic performance." Note that the italicized words represent strategies for undertaking the mission, the inclusion of which may be appropriate in some situations and may not be in others. Generally, I prefer to separate a mission (the "why") from its strategies (the "how"), but this is a point around which various viewpoints exist.

Step 7. Stimulate Community Readiness

Communicating the vision and mission is helpful for attracting the support and participation of others. After all, there will be no program if it does not go beyond the original team and council.

Community readiness is a central element to success. This term refers to the degree to which a community is adequately prepared to become involved and engaged with the program (Stith et al., 2006). To get to that point, effective coalitions need to be built and maintained between the council and community subgroups. Including representatives from important subgroups on the planning council in order to make it representative is a useful step to take.

Activities of the council and all aspects of the program to be developed need to fit the community. By community "fit," I mean, "meeting the identified needs of the community and designing interventions to be appropriate for the cultural groups targeted in the community" (Morrissey et al., 1997).

Communities can be conceptualized in terms of their readiness for change, just as individuals or organizations can. Some communities are more open to it than others. Attempting to develop a prevention program in a community that enjoys a history and culture supportive of innovation and change, of course, increases the possibility for participation, program adoption, and eventual success. The higher the resistance to change and innovation, on the other hand, the less likely it is that the prevention program will be welcomed and supported.

Therefore, assessing a community's change readiness is important to do. Several questions are useful to consider, including the following 25 that are arranged into categories of (a) context, (b) leadership, (c) collaboration, (d) cultural relevance, and (e) change attitude:

Context

1. What are the community demographics?
2. How do subgroups get along?
3. How is the community influenced by the larger environment?
4. What is the community culture (e.g., traditional/changing, open/closed)?
5. How available are community services to residents?
6. How accessible are these services?
7. What is the relationship among structures (e.g., politics, economics)?
8. How functional is the community?
9. How healthy is the community (physical, mental, economic, political, etc.)?
10. What community resources are available to support change?

Leadership

11. Can community leaders (elected, appointed, emerging, "natural") be identified?
12. What is the relationship between leaders and community residents?
13. To what degree are community leaders open to change?
14. Are there "change champions" in the community?

Collaboration

15. What community organizations have been/could be involved with change?
16. To what degree is working together present among community organizations?

Cultural Relevance

17. What are the dominant values and beliefs and the desired outcomes of community members?
18. What is the overall culture of the community and its members?
19. What are the historical patterns of functioning?
20. What cultural traditions mark this community?
21. What are the nuances of cultural evolution in the community?

Change Attitude

22. What seems to be the prevailing attitude about change in the community?

23. What is the community's history of change and innovation?

24. What are the attitudes about prevention in general?

25. What are the attitudes about the prevention issue you are considering?

LEARNING EXERCISE 7.4

Process Check #2

Conduct another process check.

How have you been doing since the last check?

What progress is being made?

How are team members feeling about their own participation and that of others?

Again, what can be done to sustain and to improve functioning?

Step 8. Assess

Community readiness is one area for assessment. It can be accomplished independently or as part of a larger local ecological assessment.

Both a local assessment and a literature review assessment need to be conducted, with one informing the other. These assessments are more rigorous than the exploration that characterized Step 2 (identify potential community issue) and Step 3 (explore relevant professional literature).

a. *Conduct a local ecological assessment.* Community interventions need to be based on a comprehensive assessment of the community. An ecological assessment permits examination of the community from various vantage points, including personal and environmental characteristics, and from multiple levels that range from the individual through the level nesting the community itself (e.g., city, state) and beyond, if appropriate. Ecological assessments, because they attend to influences of environmental and social factors (as well as those of person-centered ones), are especially relevant when conditions of poverty, class, or other unique social and economic contexts are involved (Okamoto et al., 2006; L. Smith, 2008).

Ecological assessments also allow for differing forms of assessment, including use of data produced during research (e.g., through surveys or focus group data) and previously collected and archived data (e.g., U.S. Census; Centers for Disease Control and Prevention health data). Assessments can be designed to include methods for identifying strengths and resources located within community members and the community itself. This "strengths-based" information supplies a useful counterbalance to deficit-oriented information, which typically is easier to obtain. Strengths also can serve as a starting point for building programs.

Waldo and Schwartz (2008, in Hage et al., 2007) provide a useful, ecologically based approach for considering prevention assessment and research. In their Prevention Research Matrix, they ask program planners and evaluators to think of several intersecting and interrelated issues. For example, they suggest that prevention planners consider the multicultural context surrounding the biological, psychological, and sociocultural development of the targeted population. They advocate that assessment be conducted prior to preventive intervention, with attention given to any relationships between causal and outcome factors. Identifying the prevalence (total number) of existing problems is important when intending to lower incidence (emergence of new problems).

Waldo and Schwartz point out, also, that assessment results will inform what kind of preventive intervention might be needed, given the data produced. Would it be a universal approach where all in a population are targeted? Would it be aimed at an at-risk (selective) population or at an indicated population whose members are further along in problem entrenchment (Gordon, 1983; Mrazek & Haggerty, 1994)? What sorts of research services might stem from this analysis? Dissemination of findings? Studies of impact or of cost-effectiveness? All of these? These are the kinds of factors that influence prevention planning, intervention, and research services.

b. *Search for evidence-based programs.* In an ecological assessment it also is imperative to search the professional literature for relevant programs that have demonstrated evidence of effectiveness. Both local and tested approaches are needed. Prevention program development and evaluation is not restricted to locally designed efforts or to those proven to work elsewhere. Recall the discussions in earlier chapters about evidence-based practices and the need to appropriately alter them to better fit local conditions—without diluting or eliminating the core elements of the program.

As you have seen from preceding chapters, there are a number of credible sources that can point to evidence-based programs. For instance, continuing our example that is concerned with community violence, the Center for the Study and Prevention of Violence (CSPV, 1996) contains a searchable set of violence prevention programs that have been judged as effective. In its *Blueprints for Violence Prevention* project, 11 prevention and intervention "Blueprints" programs are identified that meet a strict scientific standard of program effectiveness. These

11 programs have been found to be effective in reducing adolescent violent crime, aggression, delinquency, and substance abuse. Another 18 programs have been identified as "promising" programs. More than 600 programs have been reviewed, and the center continues to look for programs that meet the selection criteria.

Blueprint programs can be examined for potential adoption. Sometimes a program used elsewhere can fit well in a different location with a similar population. Not to beat a dead horse (too severely), but it bears repeating that, most likely, adaptation will be needed to fit the program with the local community and its members because ecologies differ across settings. A critical concern always relates to the program's cultural relevance. How will it fit the local community? What adjustments of "non-core" factors could be made to improve its cultural relevance without cutting into the "meat" of the program? How can local ecological assessment information be used to assist in that goal?

In the next chapter attention is given to the remaining two steps of the PD&E approach. These deal with preparing to implement and evaluate the prevention program. Step 9 involves constructing the specific procedures for the program and how to deliver it, while Step 10 addresses researching and evaluating it.

Summary

Prevention program development and evaluation depends on careful planning that is based on the processes of community, collaboration, and cultural relevance (the three Cs). Attending to these processes helps to lay the groundwork in the first eight steps of the PPD&E approach. These eight steps are: (a) Establish and maintain a team, (b) Identify a potential community issue, (c) Explore related professional literature, (d) Develop a germinal idea, (e) Engage stakeholders in a planning council, (f) Create a shared vision and mission, (g) Stimulate community readiness, and (h) Assess (through a local ecological assessment and a search for evidence-based programs).

You were encouraged to select your own prevention topic to work with as you become acquainted with the PPD&E steps and begin to apply them to prevention in future chapters. If, by chance, you escaped this snare, it's not too late! Just return to Learning Exercise 7.1, complete it, and move on. You will find it to be helpful.

CHAPTER 8

Designing the Prevention Program and Evaluation Plan

Steps 9–10

Designing the Prevention Plan and Evaluation

Planners have now developed a strong planning group, which we have called a planning council. This is a vital accomplishment. It is time to identify and develop what they will seek to prevent or promote.

Steps 1–8 are critically important for preparing the way for proper prevention planning and evaluation, including giving attention to collaboration, community, and cultural relevance. Steps 9 and 10 build on this preparation, guiding design of the prevention plan and its evaluation. These two steps are where the "rubber meets the road" in the entire PPD&E process. People who like to work with detail may find this step refreshing. People who don't may well find it frustrating. Nonetheless, it is very important for moving a project plan ahead because it is in these steps that concepts are translated into concrete responsibilities and timelines and judgments can result about the program's utility.

Step 9, Design the Prevention Program Plan, includes determining the problem incidence, goals to be addressed in the program, and the details of what will be done, by whom, with what resources, and in what time sequences. Step 10, Design the Prevention Program Evaluation Plan, lays out a framework for evaluation of how the plan was actually put into practice (process evaluation), and the extent to which goals were met (outcome evaluation).

Steps 9 and 10 are presented in Table 8.1.

Table 8.1   Implement and Evaluate (Steps 9–10)

STEP 9: Design the prevention program plan
STEP 10: Design the prevention program evaluation plan

Step 9: Design the Prevention Program Plan

In general, the purpose in Step 9 is to enumerate relationships among the targeted problem, goals of the program, strategies to be followed in reaching those objectives, activities within those strategies, tasks to be accomplished within each activity, resources required to fulfill the tasks, and timelines for completing the tasks, activities, and strategies. See Table 8.2, which depicts these elements.

Table 8.2   PPD&E Step 9: Design the Prevention Program Plan

a. Determine problem in general terms
b. Use adapted incidence reduction formula
c. Set objectives
d. Choose among alternative strategies
e. Plan implementation
• Objective
• Strategies
• Activities
• Tasks
• Resources
• Timelines

Key Point. It must be emphasized once again that the most significant step to take in this process is to conceptualize and define the prevention problem in terms of incidence reduction. The focus of the final two chapters is on this very topic.

In addition to the weight we will place on viewing problem identification through an incidence reduction lens, certainly all steps in the program development and evaluation sequence are important. A description of the program development and evaluation sequence follows, along with a truncated example of bullying in a university residence hall.

The general program development and evaluation sequence follows:

PROBLEM–OBJECTIVES–STRATEGIES–ACTIVITIES–
TASKS–RESOURCES–TIMELINES

For example:

INITIAL PROBLEM: Too many bullying incidents occur, leading to personal and academic difficulties. (Note: This initial problem statement will be defined in incidence reduction terms in the next chapter.)

OBJECTIVE 1: To improve communication skills by 50% among Sapler residence hall students in the prevention program, compared to the no-treatment control group.

STRATEGY 1: Half of students in Sapler residence hall participate in tested interactive communication skills training program that has been culturally adapted to fit the students and university.

ACTIVITY 1: Students participate in three-session empathy skills workshop.

TASK 1: Students learn how to identify affective statements.

RESOURCES: Four trained facilitators per classroom; materials.

TIMELINE: Workshop dates, personnel, evaluation timing all specified.

EVALUATE: Process and outcome.

Step 9a. Determine the Problem in General Terms

What is a problem? Adapted from a classic definition by Craig (1978), a problem generally can be understood as: a situation or condition of people or an environment that is considered to be undesirable. Unless something is done to change that situation or condition, the problem will continue to exist in the future. Moreover, in prevention the key is to stop problem onset or to reduce the rate of onset.

Analyzing a problem aids in understanding it and how to address it. Some important analytical questions include (Craig, 1978; Kettner, Moroney, & Martin, 2008):

- What is the nature of the situation or condition?
- How do people experience this problem?
- Whose problem is it?
- What seem to be its causes?

- What is the scope of the problem?
- How does the situation or condition fit with local values?
- Are ethnic, gender, class, or other issues of diversity involved?
- What may happen if nothing is done?

Mental health and education problems inhibit successful and satisfying functioning. These can run a broad gamut ranging across psychological and emotional disturbances (e.g., depression), negative lifestyles involving repetitive bad choices, and dysfunctional behaviors such as missing school, or violence against self or others.

Step 9b. Define the Problem in Incidence Reduction Terms

In prevention the goal is to stop or minimize undesirable, hurtful problems from emerging in the first place—or as quickly as possible, once it has progressed—through environmental change and personal change programmatic efforts. This is incidence reduction.

To capture incidence reduction, the process of problem identification needs not only to recognize but also to expand the general definition presented above, and to provide a means for assessing if problem onset has been stopped or if its rate of development has been reduced. Identifying a problem from an incidence reduction vantage point will be the entire focus of the next chapter. As well, its step-by-step process is contained in Appendix G. At this point, then, only the planning formula for prevention incidence reduction is outlined. You will recognize it from Chapter 4, where the concept was first introduced.

Incidence Reduction for Problem Identification in Prevention Program Development and Evaluation: Adapted Incidence Reduction Formula

---

Decrease: DEFICITS

Environmental Risks and Stressors: (Physical × Social × Culture)
Physical Environment: Stressors in Natural and Built Environment
Social Environment: Stressors in Informal and Formal Social Relations
Culture: Exploitation, Oppression, Underlying Values and Patterns

---

Increase: STRENGTHS

Protective Factors: (Personal × Interpersonal × Group × System)
Personal Factors: Self-Esteem, Well-Being, Resilience, Self-Efficacy
Interpersonal Factors: Interpersonal and Coping Skills, Engagement
Group Factors: Collective Efficacy, Social Support
System Factors: Ecological Competence, Advocacy

Applying this formula, *which will occur in the next two chapters,* allows for defining the problem in incidence reduction terms. In turn, this step leads to determining objectives for the prevention effort and then to all subsequent PD&E steps.

Step 9c. Set the Program Objectives

Arguably, it is important and necessary to develop objectives in life. In program development and evaluation there is little argument that this step is necessary. The following saying applies: "If you don't know where you're headed, how will you know if you've arrived?"

The relation between an objective and a problem is inverted. That is, an objective essentially is a problem tilted upside down. A simplified campus interpersonal violence example may help communicate this idea. If the problem is that certain residence hall students are bullied through pejorative name-calling, the objective might be to reduce pejorative name-calling among students in that residence hall by 50%. So, where the problem identifies a situation or condition that is *undesirable,* an objective converts the deficit into a statement of *desirability*.

Objectives stem from goals, which set an overall direction for action. Objectives are more precise than goals. The acronym SPAMO helps to define some of this precision, where an objective needs to be:

S: Specific

P: Performance based

A: Achievable

M: Measurable

O: Objective

Objectives also need to be clearly and concretely written so that anyone who reads them will be able to understand them. It is helpful, as well, to tie criteria for success to objectives that can be used to evaluate whether the program and participants were able to achieve what was set out for them.

Step 9d. Choose Among Alternative Strategies

During the earlier process in Step 4 of Lay the Groundwork (Develop a Germinal, Motivating Idea), a variety of possibilities may have emerged. Now, in the preparing-for-implementation stage, these tentative ideas can be more closely examined and evaluated. In addition, more creative idea generation can occur if that seems appropriate or needed.

The planners are now intending to formulate a strategy that seems likely to meet the objective that has been set. A strategy is a series or a group of activities that are implemented to reach the identified objective.

In the bullying example of campus interpersonal violence, the strategic issue is how—that is, by what broad methods—will name-calling be reduced by 50%? One of several possible strategies might be to create a broad bullying prevention program that would contain a specific component aimed at eliminating pejorative name-calling among residents. One of several activities within that strategy might be to form a team to plan the program. One task among many within the planning team activity might be to attain approval for the plan that is created. You can see how the planning process becomes ever more specific and concrete, progressing next to resources needed, timelines, and designation of responsibilities to persons or groups. The next section details these steps.

Step 9e. Plan How to Implement
the Prevention Program

Objectives–Strategies–Activities–Tasks–Resources–Timelines. It is helpful to create a system that can "hold" planning information, be publicly posted, and be used for program evaluation monitoring. I have found Program Evaluation and Review Technique (PERT) charting, suggested by Craig (1978), to be especially helpful for this purpose. PERT charting provides the capacity to show relationships among objectives, strategies, activities, resources, timelines, and persons/groups who will be held responsible.

PERT Chart. An example excerpt of a PERT chart is presented as Figure 8.1 on the following page. In this PERT chart, a different objective is the focus, but still related to bullying. This objective is to reduce name-calling among college students in one residence hall. The strategy is participation in a Bully Busting program. The PERT chart presents a number of activities within the strategy, when they would be offered, and by whom.

   Observe that the blocks inside the PERT chart each represent activities that, when summed, are intended to make up the strategy. In turn, the plan is structured so that the objective can be accomplished by implementing the strategy. Take a look.

Activities With a Strategy. The PERT chart example allows planners to scan at a glance a series of activities over time as well as who is responsible for completing each one. For instance, by January 15 the planning council is responsible for forming teams; by March 10 two activities are to be accomplished, one by the assessment team and the other with the community. The sum of all these activities produces the strategy, "Conduct a Bully Busting Program," which is intended to result in meeting program objectives, including "reduce name-calling by 50%." (Note: There most likely would be several objectives, each of which would have a PERT chart.)

Tasks Within an Activity. For further specification, each activity is broken down by the tasks that compose it. To each of these tasks is assigned a person(s) responsible, resources needed, and a timeline for completion. The form below depicts this process, using the example activity of "data collected" from the PERT chart.

Task Planning for One Activity			
For one activity, plan its tasks:			
Activity: Data collected by Feb. 20			
Tasks	*Who?*	*How?*	*When?*
1. Design method	Assessment team	Face-to-face meeting	Feb. 10
2. Attain approval	Planning council	E-mail correspondence	Feb. 12
3. Develop procedures	Assessment team	Face-to-face meeting	Feb. 14
4. Implement	Assessment team	Focus groups	Feb. 16
5. Organize data	Assessment team	Summarize notes	Feb. 20

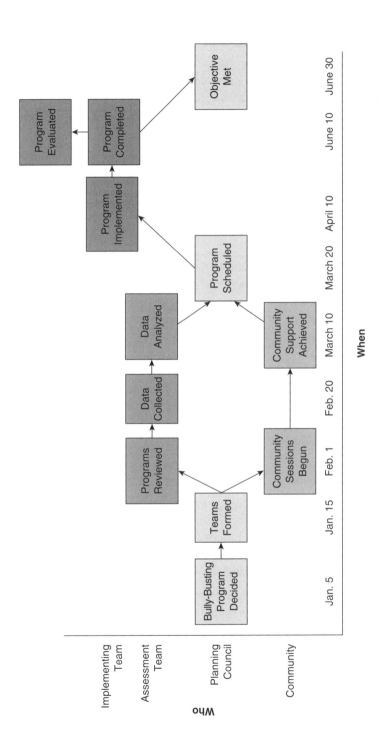

Figure 8.1 PERT Chart. Strategy Example: Bully-Busting Program

Source: © John Conyne.

Resources Needed. Activities and the tasks that compose them are analyzed for the resources needed to accomplish them. In our example of using focus groups to collect data, relatively few materials and little equipment are required. A procedure needs to be developed to record ideas generated. This might involve dedicating one person to that role who uses a laptop computer. E-mail capacity is needed to permit communicating about approval with the planning council. Meeting room space is necessary to house the face-to-face meetings. A printer to produce the summarization of organized data is needed. This is a parsimonious method.

Set Timelines. Neglecting to assign deadlines to tasks is tantamount to failure. How many times have you been part of an enthusiastic conversation that went something like: "Yes! We'll need to get this done soon," as all parties exit with high intentions but with no grasp of what "soon" means. As in the Task Planning chart above, specific timelines need to be agreed upon by all who are involved, or success is threatened.

Note that other activities and associated tasks would require more elaborate resources and much more detailed task planning. A clear example is the activity "program implementation," scheduled to occur over a 2-month period between April 10 and June 10. Implementation steps would need to be identified and assigned to personnel, with accompanying time frames and necessary resources.

From the illustration of the data collection activity that has been presented, you might be able to get a good sense of how task planning for an activity is accomplished. But to test that out, take a look at the next learning exercise.

LEARNING EXERCISE 8.1

Examining Your Own Prevention Topic

Steps 9 and 10, as I have mentioned, are the "nitty-gritty" of prevention program development and evaluation. Programs must be specifically planned with built-in procedures for monitoring and evaluating their success.

Let's return to the prevention topic you have been working with as you've been moving through all these steps. Comment below on your ability to describe in concrete terms the

Problem-Objectives-Strategies-Activities-Tasks-Resources-Timelines

Comment here:

_____

_____

_____

As you look at the relationship among all these linkages, jot notes to the following two questions:

What could go wrong with my plan?

_____

_____

_____

How could I prevent those things from going wrong?

_____

_____

_____

Step 10: Design the Prevention Program Evaluation Plan

Program evaluation planning needs to be concerned with many issues. Perhaps foremost among them is incorporating evaluation of program processes and program outcomes. Table 8.3 summarizes several elements that are useful to include when designing a program evaluation plan. Attention is given to both process and outcome evaluation issues. In addition, in the case of prevention programs, it is important that evaluation consider incidence reduction. Let's begin with process and outcome.

Step 10a. Process/Formative Evaluation: How Did the Program Work?

Process (formative) evaluation is conducted by monitoring program implementation and providing ongoing feedback to program planners. This feedback can then be used to make adjustments necessary to keep the program on course, to be responsive to changing demands, or to take advantage of new opportunities. PERT charts and task accomplishment plans, such as those illustrated above, are helpful for keeping track of planned events and for examining and documenting the fidelity of how the program components are actually being implemented in relation to the plan. These often are discordant, for many reasons. The main point is that the real world never conforms to how we have envisioned it. There always will be deviations. A discrepancy analysis can assist in detecting gaps and, if timely enough and otherwise feasible, can guide positive changes. Making

Table 8.3   PPD&E Step 10: Design the Prevention Program Evaluation Plan

a. Process/formative evaluation
Key prevention processes: • Context considered • Community orientation • Cultural relevance/fit • Collaboration/partnerships • Fidelity • Guided adaptability • Evidence based
b. Outcome/summative evaluation
Key prevention questions: • Were new cases eliminated or diminished? • Were deficits reduced? • Was the environment improved? • Were strengths and natural supports increased? Key prevention criteria: • Adequacy, appropriateness • Effectiveness, efficiency • Side effects, sustainability • Transferability, dissemination • Usefulness and general contribution

necessary adaptations allows the program to fit dynamic situations more closely and appropriately.

In terms of those evaluation criteria we considered in Table 8.3, maintaining both program "fidelity" and "fit" is important. Process evaluation is concerned with the context (C), for example, shifting or stable environmental conditions; appropriateness (A), for example, cultural relevance and fit; adequacy (A), for example, sufficiency of resources; efficiency (E), for example, cost-benefit of people served in relation to costs of the program being implemented; and the effort (E) expended, for example, hours of delivery time.

Step 10b. Outcome/Summative Evaluation: How About Results?

This large topic relates to four major considerations: local effects of the program, including considerations related to incidence reduction; sustainability; replication and transferability; and dissemination.

Local Effects of the Program. Local effects, including incidence reduction, are of high importance. All evaluation criteria are important with outcome or summative evaluation. The primary criterion, however, is effectiveness. Did the prevention program reach its stated goals? Moreover, while a prevention program certainly can be effective without showing incidence reduction, as I've pointed out, incidence reduction is the ultimate goal. Prevention programs need to be evaluated for numerous outcomes, including if new cases of problems diminished as a result of the prevention program.

Some of the many important summative evaluation questions include:

- Did the program reach its goals?
- Were new cases eliminated or diminished (incidence reduction)?
- Were deficits reduced?
- Was the environment improved?
- Were strengths and natural supports increased?
- Did the program make the difference it set out to make in participants?

In our overly simplified example, was name-calling reduced by 50% among residents after the prevention program was introduced? This question runs to incidence reduction if it also can be shown that students new to the residence hall who in the past might have been at risk for being called derogatory names did not experience this form of bullying following completion of the prevention program. An even more clear demonstration of incidence reduction in this example would compare two residence halls with similar name-calling prevalence, one of which would receive the prevention treatment while the other would not. Comparing the two halls for baseline prevalence of name-calling just prior to the start of the program and at its conclusion would permit conclusions to be drawn about incidence reduction. In the best of all worlds, the number of new cases of name-calling (incidence) in the prevention residence hall would be significantly lower than in the comparison hall not participating in the prevention program.

To be able to demonstrate bottom-line effects, the prevention program needs to be set within the best research design possible for the circumstances. Community conditions often are not amenable to scientific research designs, of course. Still, program planners should aspire to use the classic research design of randomized experimental-control with established measures whenever possible. Sometimes this is possible; often it is not for many reasons. But always start there; shoot for it. Examine research and evaluation designs of "model" programs that have been able to demonstrate evidence of success for ideas of how to begin producing the best possible design for your situation. Scale down to the next best design, then the next best, as conditions warrant. Qualitative designs emphasizing careful description will not be able to generalize beyond the local setting but, depending on what is asked, these studies can reveal substantive information about how a particular program worked, how participants experienced the activities, and how they evolved. In fact, sometimes a qualitative design may best fit a particular situation. Combinations of quantitative and qualitative research designs can sometimes reflect the best of both worlds.

LEARNING EXERCISE 8.2

Defining Process and Outcome Evaluation

Process (or formative evaluation) and outcome (or summative evaluation) are both important in program evaluation.

What is process evaluation?

Provide a definition with two examples of *process.*

Definition:

_____

_____

Example 1:

_____

_____

Example 2:

_____

_____

What is outcome evaluation?

Give a definition with two examples of *outcomes.*

Definition:

_____

_____

Example 1:

_____

_____

Example 2:

_____

_____

Take your own prevention topic. How would you incorporate attention to process and to outcome?

_____

_____

Sustainability. Sustainability of effects realized is an essential outcome matter. Effectiveness data are very important, but they do not tell the whole story. If the program demonstrates immediate positive effects, compared with control, that is most welcomed. Rejoice! However, will these effects last over time? In this case, will the lessened frequency of name-calling remain? What plans have been made to extend effects, to enable participants to attain the necessary support and encouragement to maintain their gains? Sometimes, as pointed out earlier, booster sessions can be helpful in prolonging learning and change. In terms of measurement, research designs can be established to include longer term follow-up. And consideration needs to be given to creating programs and research designs that are longitudinal in scope, being able to endure over time.

Replication and Transferability. The next outcome issues are replication, transferability, and usefulness. Indeed, if the program is deemed effective and sustainable, others should benefit from it, as well. Therefore, is the program described in enough detail that it could be implemented again (replicated) or be transferred for use in similar circumstances by others? Imagine the program being parachuted down into another setting. What are the chances it could be implemented there? Would people there understand it? Is there enough information provided so they could move ahead with adoption or, more likely, with adaptation? Program personnel need to describe their interventions and outcomes in sufficient detail so that others could readily understand and use them.

Dissemination. Dissemination of program processes and outcomes is a critically important issue deserving close consideration. Program personnel have an obligation to spread effective interventions. Related to transferability, above, dissemination is a step too few program personnel take. Once a program is finished and a report is filed, the norm is that not much else may occur. This kind of "program abandonment" is a pity, and it needs to change. Outcome evaluation should naturally include a dissemination phase, not just in funded projects but in all projects, where others can access program design, processes, outcomes, data, and recommendations. In this way, the storehouse of knowledge can be shared and expanded, leading to improved research and practice.

Dissemination connects directly with the scientific community. Effective and noneffective programs, as well, need to be published and presented in scientific outlets. The test might be if the science was done well. Statistically significant results are an important index of effectiveness. Yet, as pointed out earlier, clinical significance (or practical significance outside the clinical domain) also is important. We have much to learn from such projects.

Dissemination needs to be connected more closely with the practice community. Reliance on scientific publications and presentations will not reach most professional practitioners and hardly any other community workers. Efforts need to be conducted to disseminate, which often may mean to translate, program findings and procedures into local settings.

Summary

PD&E is vitally important for moving prevention from conceptual theory to practical application. In this chapter, you were introduced to a range of material and perspectives related to PD&E, centered on essential criteria (context, appropriateness, adequacy, effectiveness, efficiency, side effects, and sustainability) that are broadly applicable for both evaluating and developing programs. A general 10-step PD&E approach evolved, which includes specific attention to community-level and culturally relevant foci. "Nitty-gritty" planning and evaluation steps were summarized to complete this introductory coverage of PD&E. A simplified example of campus interpersonal violence involving bullying was used for explanatory purposes.

The importance of defining a prevention problem from an incidence reduction approach was underscored, but not fully developed in this chapter, in favor of discussing the entire sequence at this point. It will become the focus of the next two chapters.

CHAPTER 9

Back to the Future

Applying Incidence Reduction to Problem Identification in Prevention Program Development and Evaluation

Chapter Overview

- Back to the Future: Problem Identification and Prevention
- Prevention Stakes Out a Unique Path
- Problem Identification in PPD&E
- I. Contributions to Environmental Deficits (Numerator Factors)
- Learning Exercise 9.1. Process Check #3
- II. Contributions to Personal, Interpersonal, Group, and System Strengths (Denominator Factors)
- Learning Exercise 9.2. Process Check #4
- Summary

Back to the Future: Problem Identification and Prevention

Now that you've read about the complete sequence of prevention program development and evaluation, let's take a trip "back to the future" to the critically important program design step of problem identification. You read in Chapter 8 about a general definition of a problem and the importance of problem definition to program development and evaluation. It also was pointed out that in *prevention* program development and evaluation, the problem needs also to be understood in terms of incidence reduction—that is the unique path of prevention.

Prevention Stakes Out a Unique Path

Program development and evaluation in prevention needs to concern itself not only with problem reduction and strength enhancement but also with lessening the frequency of new cases of the problem or disorder. Therefore, although prevention holds much in common with all forms of help-giving, it also stakes out its own direction.

To reiterate, the key point in prevention program development and evaluation occurs at problem identification. Indeed, this early step is a critical one in all program development processes, and many scholars have tagged problem identification as the most essential and difficult step of all. When prevention is involved, that opinion is reinforced due to the unique mission of prevention programs—to lower incidence whenever possible.

In this chapter specific attention will be given to exploring the general problem of campus interpersonal violence (of which bullying, which we considered last chapter, is a part) from an incidence reduction perspective. Doing so then guides subsequent program development and evaluation steps in prevention. Follow along and also apply this approach to your own prevention topic.

Problem Identification in PPD&E

Step 9b: Identify the Problem From an Incidence Reduction Perspective

(Note: This step is in addition to the general problem definition Step 9a in Chapter 8.)

We have been considering the general problem of interpersonal violence occurring at the college level, last looking at a subset of it, bullying. At the point of identifying a problem, though, planners need to avoid becoming too specific too quickly, either in terms of identifying the problem to be addressed or how it should be solved. So, let's return to the wider issue of campus interpersonal violence, without tying it to bullying or to any other specifics at this point, and analyze it using the adapted incidence reduction formula.

We will systematically proceed through the formula's components—discussed in earlier chapters—by applying them in a general way to campus interpersonal violence. A review of each component will be followed by many questions that are intended to demonstrate how problem exploration and identification might proceed from an incidence reduction vantage point. *Once again, I encourage you also to follow through with your own prevention topic.*

Let's begin by grounding our understanding of interpersonal violence. It includes

violence between individuals, and is subdivided into family and intimate part-ner violence and community violence. The former category includes child maltreatment; intimate partner violence; and elder abuse, while the latter is broken down into acquaintance *and* stranger violence and includes youth vio-lence; assault by strangers; violence related to property crimes; and violence in workplaces and other institutions. (Violence Prevention Alliance, 2008)

It also should be pointed out that interpersonal violence includes psychological intimidation, harassment, and relational violence, forms that are particularly rele-vant to campus interpersonal violence.

Now to the general application of the adapted incidence reduction formula to problem identification. To keep the formula in front of us, it is:

Adapted Incidence Reduction Formula for Problem Identification in Prevention Program Development and Evaluation

---

Decrease: DEFICITS
　　　　　Environmental Risks and Stressors: (Physical × Social × Culture)
　　　　　Physical Environment: Stressors in Natural and Built Environment
　　　　　Social Environment: Stressors in Informal and Formal Social Relations
　　　　　Culture: Exploitation, Oppression, Underlying Values and Patterns

---

Increase: STRENGTHS
　　　　　Protective Factors: (Personal × Interpersonal × Group × System)
　　　　　Personal Factors: Self-Esteem, Well-Being, Resilience, Self-Efficacy
　　　　　Interpersonal Factors: Interpersonal and Coping Skills, Engagement
　　　　　Group Factors: Collective Efficacy, Social Support
　　　　　System Factors: Ecological Competence, Advocacy

I. Contributions to Environmental Deficits (Numerator Factors)

Reduce Environmental Deficits

Physical Environment Stressors

A. What *Physical Environmental Stressors* (natural and built environment, context, events, circumstances, situations) affect the lives of people in this population?

　(1) *What organic physical, mental, or emotional behaviors are affected by physical environmental stressors? (e.g., Down syndrome, lead poison-ing, depression, obesity, attention deficit, alcoholism)*

Students with special needs are increasing in numbers on college campuses. Figures reported by the National Center for Educational Statistics (2003–2004) showed that 11% of college students had a disability, with 22% of those disabilities accounted for by mental illness or depression.

Some of these special needs result from organic factors, in combination with external ones. It is an unfortunate circumstance that students who look or behave differently from the mainstream are at heightened vulnerability to interpersonal violence of some form. Students with physical (e.g., speech impairments, cerebral palsy, Tourette syndrome) or mental disabilities (e.g., depression, hyperactivity) may be increasingly susceptible to harassment by insensitive students. As well, students who represent diversity by virtue of race, ethnicity, age, and sexual orientation may be at higher risk. Those who are predisposed to substance abuse carry a heightened exposure to certain forms of interpersonal violence, either as victim or perpetrator. Finally, those who are particularly attractive physically, especially female students, may be at elevated risk in certain situations, such as parties involving alcohol.

(2) *How do they inhibit functioning, and what is their strength?*

To what degree are students with genetically caused disabilities or differences the subject of any form of interpersonal violence on campus? Developing a database to identify the incidence of attacks or insults might assist in answering this question.

(3) *What physical stressors are present that could affect any in the population?*

To what degree do physical elements on campus affect those with disabilities or those who possess characteristics that might serve to make them different? For example, sections of campus that may be unlit or underlit at night may present danger, or security provisions may be lax in residence halls. Or existing steps and hills may pose significant barriers for those who are physically impaired.

(4) *How could physical stressors be reduced by population members and/or by preventive intervention?*

In one case in which I was involved, we documented through campus environmental assessment that the campus quadrangle at night was perceived by many students, especially by those possessing some form of uniqueness, to be unsafe. Indeed, an elevated number of physical attacks had occurred in this space during the evening in recent weeks. A successful preventive intervention was launched by counseling center staff, guided by environmental assessment data, to advocate with central administration for increased campus lighting in that area. Once installed, physical assaults dramatically decreased (Conyne, 1975, 1978; Conyne & Clack, 1981).

Social Environment Stressors

B. What *Social Environmental Stressors* exist that can lead to psychological and emotional disorders?

In the UNESCO Declaration on the Elimination of Violence Against Women, violence against women is defined as:

> Any act of gender-based violence that results in, or is likely to result in, physical, sexual or psychological harm or suffering to women, including threats of such acts, coercion or arbitrary deprivation of liberty, whether occurring in public or private life. (UNESCO, 1993)

I present the definition above, specific to women, because its elements speak directly to the kinds of social environmental stressors that represent interpersonal violence. Threats, intimidation, harassment, coercion, exploitation, oppression, sneers, and the creation of a hostile living, classroom, or campus environment—these, and more, are aggressive social psychological forces of violence.

The following anecdote is not intended to offend anyone, but I tip you off that it is a bit raw. I include it because it's a powerful example of sexual harassment. Decades ago I sat in a classroom where the professor was located at the bottom of the room, with student seats elevated in circular rows above him. If you get the picture, he then looked up at students as he lectured. I will never forget it when he singled out a female student seated in a middle row and admonished her by name (changed here), and with an intimidating flourish—"Miss Jones, would you *kindly* close the gates of hell." I doubt that anything this outrageously hostile would ever be said today (at least, I sincerely hope not), but—once again—I cite it to highlight what is meant by a hostile social environment factor.

In those days (early 1960s) there were no campus sexual harassment policies. Today, should something of that sort occur, a student would have recourse. In this case, however, little was possible and the student was left being singled out and embarrassed, at the very least. Victims of psychological harassment, especially if it is continuous, can be greatly harmed. They may suffer from physical ailments, irritability, anxiety, nervousness, insomnia, stress, fatigue, depressive states, burnout, and in some cases suicide. Of course, the degree to which social environment stressors contribute to interpersonal violence on any one campus needs to be assessed specifically.

Students generally are resilient, able to find ways to manage in the face of external stressors. Students learn to ignore, to avoid, to team up with others, and in some cases they report perpetrators. These students will get by, but shouldn't have to be subjected to harassment.

Other students are not so skillful or sometimes not so lucky. Their coping skills and resources may be insufficient. They may not know how to develop social support. They may be unaware of reporting mechanisms or be reluctant to use them. They may have been taken advantage of in a moment of special vulnerability. These are the students who need targeted assistance.

(1) *What could be done by population members and/or by preventive intervention to reduce negative effects of the social environment?*

How noxious is the campus social environment? How toxic is the larger environment surrounding the campus? In turn, how nourishing are these environments?

What makes them so? What is the climate like? Is it supportive of students and staff who are "different"? Is a broad range of opportunities made available for students to engage in outside of classes? Are policies and procedures in place that support and protect diversity and justice? Do programs exist to assist students to establish relationships with others, to obtain counseling and advice, to provide services to students of different cultures, religions, and sexual orientations? Do minority group members have advocacy offices on campus? Is there a "campus buddy system," or its equivalent, available for nighttime walking across campus? Is the campus judicial system effective and appropriate? Does the administration take a proactive, preventive approach to education and providing care? Are advising, career development, and placement services linked and made available and accessible to students so they can better link their academic preparation with future educational and/or career application? How do faculty generally interact with students in and out of the classroom? Is the campus security system functioning effectively and with fairness, and is it ready to handle everyday occurrences and any crises that may occur? To what degree do all students feel treated like a person on campus and not just as a number or a member of a category? How do residential and Greek (if one exists) systems function in relation to student life?

(2) *How can negative behaviors be reduced?*

Do students have access to counseling, advising, and health services? Is an effective orientation and advising set of services available that can help students to learn of campus and neighboring resources that are available to them? Are counseling services comprehensive in scope, including outreach and prevention services to help students avoid problems and enhance their skills? Do students take care of themselves? Do they generally get enough rest, avoid excesses, connect with one another, stay in reasonable contact with their families, and take advantage of existing resources? Are students encouraged to balance their lives at college; to eat well; to study and prepare for classes, exams, and projects; and to form friendships? To what extent are students engaging with the campus resources that are available to them? As I mentioned earlier in this book, engagement and active involvement with positive environmental resources are critically important to healthy functioning.

Cultural Stressors in the Environment

C. What is there about the environmental *Culture* that may support exploitation and affect the lives of people in this population?

What is the dominant campus culture? What are its underlying patterns and values? The term *culture* generally refers to a complex whole, incorporating custom, law, belief, values, morals, and habits, that is learned, followed, and transmitted to future generations (Stein & Rowe, 1989). It's a tool that can define reality for members (Kagawa-Singer & Chung, 1994), indicating what is acceptable and not (Slonim, 1991). Fenichel (1989) observed, however, that culture provides a kind of framework in a social system from which people can choose. Huff and Kline's (1999) discussion of culture, which emphasizes views and practices about health, is especially pertinent to our focus on mental health prevention.

Contemporary college and university campuses reflect general society and, increasingly, the world itself. Once a bastion of the white upper and middle class, today's American higher education is a mosaic comprising many racial and ethnic groups, students from many international countries, varying socioeconomic levels, differing educational preparation, and a gender makeup whose majority now is female. College environments, therefore, are teeming entities that are full of life, change, challenge, and opportunity.

Increasingly, college campuses (as well as other educational and work settings) have been the site for wanton violence. Virginia Tech University and Northern Illinois University afford two situations that have captured the headlines due to the extreme violence that occurred on those campuses. That these events have occurred, though, is not to suggest that college campuses are violent places. In fact, they are generally quite safe.

Yet a campus culture that is embracing of all its members, whatever their own cultural background, and one that also is able to project and sustain a set of expectations, rules, and norms that support a safe and healthy environment for all is not an easy proposition to achieve and sustain. Chinks in the cultural armor inevitably occur.

(1) *Identify any abuse: Oppression? Exploitation? Marginalization? Violence?*

Often these chinks in the cultural armor are traceable to oppression and exploitation of at-risk members and to related interpersonal violence, both subtle and overt. How are students and staff from differing backgrounds regarded in the campus culture? To what degree are differences accepted, embraced, ignored, or rejected? How is diversity of thought and opinion typically handled in the class-room, on the residence floor, in the fraternity and sorority, and when walking across the quad? Is there a sense of school pride, a connection with the college or university, and a sense of community? How do people treat each other? To what degree do microaggressions, those smaller but insidious personal insults and assaults, occur? To what degree is concern shown and a sense of empathy for others demonstrated? How competitive is the culture? How supportive is it? How open is the administration to listening to students, faculty, and staff? How are "town-gown" relations? How do students generally think about having a good time? To what degree do alcohol and other drugs dominate social activities? How often do students binge-drink? How does the campus culture comply with or reject excessive drinking? Are minority cultures supported? What happens when anyone is threat-ened at the college? How safe do female students feel when walking the campus at day and at night? What populations seem to be most at risk? Why?

(2) *Describe how any oppression and exploitation are expressed in terms of ethnicity, race, gender, sexual orientation, age, religious orientation, spir-itual affiliation, socioeconomic status, and physical/mental ability.*

Oppression—the unjust or cruel use of power or authority—can be thought of as a form of interpersonal violence. So can exploitation—taking advantage of others for one's own gain. These virulent forms of interpersonal violence can be expressed quietly through institutionalized policies and procedures and through ongoing microaggressions and verbal and nonverbal slights. Or they can be expressed loudly, through specific acts of aggression against persons and property.

(3) *How could this oppression and exploitation be reduced by population members and/or by preventive intervention?*

Being oppressed or exploited are heavy burdens to bear, leaving one to feel excluded and unwanted without access to the means for changing the oppressive situation. Ongoing assessment of campus cultures for their degree of openness or closedness, their acceptance or rejection of differences, and the degree to which all members report feeling a part of the mainstream is an essential strategy for reducing interpersonal violence.

LEARNING EXERCISE 9.1

Process Check #3

As is our custom, it is a good time to conduct another process check as you (and your team, if you are fortunate) apply the adapted incidence reduction formula to identifying your problem area more specifically.

- Describe how your work is going.

  _____
  _____
  _____

- How are you working together?

  _____
  _____
  _____

- What progress are you making?

  _____
  _____
  _____

> - Are you able to gain increased understanding of how deficits are involved in the problem? Yes or No.
>
> Elaborate on your answer:
>
> _____
>
> _____
>
> _____
>
> It also is time to think ahead. What are you learning that you can transfer to your work as a preventionist?

II. Contributions to Personal, Interpersonal, Group, and System Strengths (Denominator Factors)

Increase Protective Strengths

Personal Strengths

D. How is *Self-Esteem* evidenced?

Self-esteem is the evaluative aspect of self-concept, corresponding to one's self-view as being good or bad, worthy or unworthy (Heatherton & Wyland, 2003). Bolstered self-esteem is an important building block of positive mental health (Branden, 1994). Students who feel good about themselves (but not excessively good, which can be a detriment; see Baumeister, 1998) are better able to manage their lives and to adapt effectively to changing conditions and to negative events. They also tend to interact socially and to perceive that they are valued by others. Self-esteem is associated with enjoyment, happiness, satisfaction, and success. Those who possess a positive and realistic self-esteem are less likely to engage in interpersonal violence.

(1) *What competencies tend to be shown?*

Students with positive self-esteem are more likely to think of themselves as having worth, being confident, being comfortable in meeting others, able to perform, and satisfied with their lives. They are less likely to think of themselves as being inferior to others, to feel anxious, to worry, or to be uncomfortable in new situations.

Students with a realistically positive sense of self-esteem are more likely to behave with surety in novel situations and to be optimistic and caring in their approach to others. They are less likely to be rejected and to reject others and to feel socially anxious.

To what degree are students in the targeted population evidencing these characteristics, and how might they be incorporated in a campus interpersonal violence prevention program?

(2) *What could be done by population members and/or by preventive intervention to enhance self-esteem?*

Being connected positively with others aids the development and maintenance of self-esteem. Families, friends, social organizations, group activities—all these can contribute to a bolstered self-esteem. Becoming involved in tasks that are interesting, challenging, and accomplishable also can facilitate self-esteem. Maintaining one's health, exercising, eating nutritiously, and keeping up with the demands of daily life also are important. Self-esteem is both the beneficiary of these kinds of involvements and a causal contributor to initiating and maintaining them in the first place.

Prevention programs can be constructed to give support and to enhance self-esteem in participants. Assessing levels of self-esteem is possible (e.g., Revised Janis and Field Scale; see Fleming & Courtney, 1984), followed by incorporating esteem-building activities intentionally within the program.

E. How is *Well-Being* evidenced?

Well-being is a central concept in positive psychology. It captures several inter-related components (Ryff, 1989), including self-acceptance, personal growth, purpose of life, environmental mastery, autonomy, and positive relations with others. In turn, these six components can be organized within three dominant elements of well-being: (a) psychological, (b) social, and (c) emotional. Keyes (Keyes & Lopez, 2002) further distinguishes levels of well-being between those who are flourishing (i.e., no mental illness and high levels of psychological, social, and emotional well-being) and those who are languishing (i.e., no mental illness but low levels of well-being).

Students who possess high versus low levels of well-being tend to be happier and more satisfied, hold more positive attitudes toward others, and are more likely to be connected with others and make social contributions. They also tend to possess internal and external strengths and virtues that allow them to engage more productively in the world. These students would be less likely to commit subtle or overt forms of interpersonal violence.

(1) *What competencies tend to be shown?*

Students with high levels of well-being are likely to demonstrate ecological competency, autonomy, positive relations with others, self-acceptance, personal growth, a purpose in life, social acceptance, positive affect, a sense of coherence, happiness, and life satisfaction. These competencies, or human strengths, are thought to be the "active ingredients of positive living" (Snyder & Lopez, 2007, p. 73).

To what degree are students in the targeted population evidencing these characteristics, and how might they be incorporated in a campus interpersonal violence prevention program?

(2) *What could be done by population members and/or by preventive intervention to enhance well-being?*

A number of accessible assessment scales have been made available online. An example is the Values in Action Strengths Scale, VIA-IS, at www.positivepsychology.org. This Web site includes a range of resources. Individuals can access these, complete the scales, and receive and analyze their profiles. Moreover, a number of exercises have been created to assist in identifying and enhancing strengths. For instance, a person can pick 1 of their 10 main strengths and try using that strength five times a day for 5 days. Such attempts have been shown to both augment the strength and foster a habit to use it more frequently. Other strength-building exercises have been developed in areas such as forgiveness, altruism, and gratitude.

Prevention programs also can be designed to activate the psychological, social, and emotional well-being domains of participants. For example, a mentoring program can develop strengths in the mentor (e.g., in altruistic behavior, or in social coherence) just as in the mentee. Interpersonal violence prevention programs that incorporate attention to supporting and enhancing well-being contribute to a healthy foundation for participants, the benefits of which can radiate across many situations.

F. How is *Resilience* evidenced?

People "bounce back" more often than not. Most college students—but certainly not all of them—are in the "bloom of life" and are more likely than not to show resilience. That is, they tend to be positively adaptive in the face of significant risk to return to a relative state of typical functioning for them (Masten & Reed, 2002). As well, resilience tends to dampen the need to strike back and to inflict revenge, both of which are aspects of interpersonal violence. The reservoir of strength and experience that allows for resilience to occur is an important factor in prevention programming.

(1) *What competencies tend to be shown?*

Positive attitudes and behaviors associated with and promoting resilience include: having positive self-perceptions, being self-efficacious, holding a positive outlook about life, possessing a good sense of humor, being generally appealing to others, having a purpose in life, maintaining close relationships, being connected to positive peers, and being involved in organized and effective settings (Masten & Reed, 2002). To what degree are students in the targeted population evidencing these characteristics, and how might they be incorporated in a campus interpersonal violence prevention program?

(2) *What could be done by population members and/or by preventive intervention to enhance their resilience?*

Masten and Reed (2002) have identified a number of strategies that can promote resilience. These include preventing risk and stressors (e.g., reduce drinking, smoking, and drug use), developing assets (e.g., provide recreational opportunities), and mobilizing human systems (e.g., teach effective coping strategies). Colleges and universities can be intentionally designed as positive socializing systems through providing resilience and strengths-development programming (Lopez, Janowski, & Wells, 2005). Such approaches can help students resist risk, and draw from their strengths to promote concord and a sense of community.

G. How is *Self-Efficacy* evidenced?

Self-efficacy refers to a person's capacity to produce effects because of his or her own actions (Bandura, 1997). Self-efficacy develops over time, it is learned, and it can be taught. It is a social cognition theory rooted in the tenet that people can actively shape their lives instead of being controlled by environmental forces.

Self-efficacy has been found to be influential in a range of psychological problems. It can exert a protective role against maladies, and it also can be used to empower people to become proactive agents.

As disaster mental health volunteers for the American Red Cross, we are encouraged to assist those affected by disasters (e.g., hurricanes, tornadoes, fires) to identify once again their capacity for self-efficacy and positive coping. This is no place for therapy. Engaging in problem-solving strategies, mental health volunteers provide support, and they help residents of temporary shelters, for instance, to recall what has worked in the past that might be useful in their present situation. As many of those affected are normal folks overcome for the moment by adverse circumstances, this positive approach often finds some success. (Of course, deeper forms of trauma require additional forms of intervention.) Generally, though, people need some guidance in rediscovering what they already do well and what usually works, and to reaffirm their belief that they can persevere, get support, and come out of this crisis, too.

(1) *What competencies tend to be shown?*

Self-efficacy involves people thinking their way through a problem and then acting on it. They envision what they have done that's worked in other similar situations, observe others who are moving ahead effectively in the situation, imagine themselves positively handling the situation, indicate to themselves that they can do it, and then move ahead by acting on that belief. As you can see, problem solving is intermeshed throughout this sequence, combined with a hopeful attitude.

The degree to which self-efficacy is evidenced by target population members, and how this quality could be further developed, is a salient issue for designing prevention programs.

(2) *What could be done by population individuals and/or by preventive intervention to enhance their sense of personal self-efficacy?*

Learning self-efficacy principles is possible through self-education and certainly through the guidance of an expert, such as in training workshops or in psychotherapy. Prevention programs often include self-efficacy training; some programs feature it. Self-efficacy runs through positive psychology and social-emotional training in such domains as self-control, emotional understanding, positive self-esteem, relationship development, and interpersonal problem solving.

Interpersonal Strengths

Interpersonal strengths build on personal strengths. They refer to our abilities to relate, work, and play with others. Because humans are interpersonal beings and much of our lives are spent in the company of others, being interpersonally competent is essential to healthy functioning. In turn, interpersonal competence is a potent antidote to interpersonal violence.

H. How are *Interpersonal and Coping Skills* evidenced?

College students are likely to possess higher than average interpersonal and coping skills. Yet some students fall outside this generality, finding interpersonal situations anxiety producing or unfulfilling. In more extreme cases, those students who wall themselves off from others by consistently choosing isolation may be at heightened risk for psychological dysfunction. At the least, they might trigger concern that should be explored judiciously.

In any case, positive interpersonal and coping skills contribute strongly to successful and satisfying living. Students with such skills generally are able to connect with others, find their way through the university system effectively, negotiate challenges they face, move ahead with plans, and respond well to disruptions.

(1) *What competencies tend to be shown?*

Interpersonal Skills. Students with well-developed interpersonal skills show the capacity to communicate effectively with others. They can listen, speak clearly, and start and maintain conversations, and they show respect and empathy toward others. Their good social skills also allow them to participate socially, to converse with those who may be potential dates, and to develop and maintain relationships. They can be assertive in situations that call for it, and can distinguish generally between arguing and debating. They are able to problem-solve and to make decisions adequately. They take in information, relate it to their own values and principles, weigh evidence, and produce alternatives. They can connect with others when needed and find private space when desired.

Coping Skills. In addition to the above interpersonal skills, those who are able to cope well can stop action when needed to get a "breather." They can relax, breathe deeply, meditate, or use other strategies for relieving tension. They can seek support and assistance from others when that may be helpful or necessary. They have learned how to think through a problem, to control emotional overreaction to situations, and to negotiate with others when differences occur, and they have found ways to deal with anxiety and crises.

Therefore, in defining the problem to be addressed, it is important to assess the degree to which the target population members possess and use adequate interpersonal and coping skills and how these could be enhanced as part of a campus interpersonal violence prevention program.

> (2) *What could be done by population members and/or by preventive intervention to enhance their interpersonal skills?*

Life experience enables many students to develop skills that are productive and helpful. Some students can benefit from counseling to help develop a richer and more effective repertoire of interpersonal and coping skills. Psychoeducation and counseling groups can be especially useful for them. Prevention programs are particularly powerful when they catalyze the interpersonal and coping skills of participants, or when they build on existing strengths. The substance abuse prevention work of Botvin and associates, beginning with their award-winning program (Botvin & Tortu, 1988), consistently incorporates several sessions of what they term "life skills training," including social skills, decision making, coping skills, and so on.

As with all other areas included within this incidence reduction formula, assessing the degree to which relevant factors are present or absent in a target population is recommended, with results serving to guide next steps.

I. How is *Engagement* evidenced?

You may recall the Ruby and Oren story from earlier, where weekly card-playing games weren't the main event for them but getting together with their friends to do it was. Active engagement with others is a vital interpersonal strength to possess. Out of this interaction can come much of value, not the least of which is fun, enjoyment, and a sense of coherence. Moreover, "friends can be good medicine," as a California prevention program of the 1970s indicated, for through friends (and family) we learn, get and give support, and feel connected.

Engagement, although I've labeled it as an interpersonal strength, also can be found in nonhuman situations. For instance, I tend to become totally engaged while writing. Seconds, minutes, hours can pass without any notice. Csikszentmihalyi (1990), as I mentioned before, called this a state of "flow." My friend Bill Caddoo can spend hours on end moving earth with what he calls his many earth-moving "toys" (bulldozers and backhoes, for example), perfectly happy to be at play in that way. Fully engaged. Others can surf, fly, read, see clients, and the list goes on. Having resources, knowledge, and skills is not enough. The trick is to find something you like, can do, and that doesn't hurt anyone—and then begin.

> (1) *What competencies tend to be shown?*

When actively engaged, any tendency toward self-absorption is put on hold. Anxieties are given a rest. Boredom is an unknown experience. Time seems to lose relevance. An actively engaged person is connecting with something larger, and all seems well with the world.

To what degree are students in the targeted population evidencing these characteristics, and how might they be incorporated in a campus interpersonal violence prevention program?

> (2) *What could be done by population members and/or by preventive intervention to enhance their ability to become engaged?*

Nancy Tobler's (2000) three large meta-analyses of drug prevention programs clearly show that small, interactive programs produce a higher average effectiveness than noninteractive ones. These interactive programs include attention to coping skills, stress reduction, goal setting, and decision making and problem solving. When delivered interactively, increased gains were realized. Forms of interaction included having everyone actively involved through such means as peer participation, peer modeling, role plays that are student generated, and rehearsal of drug refusal skills.

This process of active interaction is associated with active engagement. Passive listening, lectures, teacher-centered class discussions, and unstructured sessions all were found wanting in her analyses. What works in life is what works in prevention programming: become actively involved and, likewise, find ways to get people in prevention programs actively involved.

Group Strengths

Group strengths emerge from the interactive dynamics of individuals who make up the group. Interactions are multiplicative and powerful. Take a small group of size 5, for instance. Considering pairings alone, 10 possibilities emerge. In a group of size 12, 66 pairs are possible. (To compute these pairings, use this formula: $[N \times (N - 1)]/2$.) Of course, other interactions occur in addition to pairs, such as those among three and four members. The sum of all these interactions, if properly coordinated, yields a dynamic property far exceeding what might result from single factors added sequentially.

Groups, collectives, and populations are especially important in prevention programming due to their potential power and to the very definition of prevention itself. You will recall that prevention is intended to forestall the development of new problems in large numbers of people.

Prevention program assessment during problem identification needs to incorporate the group level. What is the target group capable of? What are its strengths, and how can they be catalyzed and magnified?

J. How is *Collective Efficacy* evidenced?

Just as individuals can learn to gain increased control over their life events by applying principles of self-efficacy, it is possible for large numbers of people—collectives—to mobilize, collaborate, and pursue shared objectives. Collective efficacy, as defined by Bandura (1997), is the degree to which people believe they can work together effectively to accomplish goals they hold in common. Collective efficacy is a group strength and results from members' beliefs that their interactive and coordinative dynamics can "create an emergent property that is more than the sum of the individual attributes" (pp. 477–478).

Assessing collective efficacy is challenging because it is difficult to separate individual- from group-level beliefs, and few measures currently exist. Bandura points out that two means are available. The first results from aggregating individual members' appraisals of what their individual capabilities are in the group. The second involves summing their appraisals of the group's capabilities as a whole.

To what degree are students in the targeted population evidencing these characteristics, and how might they be incorporated in a campus interpersonal violence prevention program?

What could be done by population group members and/or by preventive intervention to enhance their sense of collective efficacy?

Prevention planners can stimulate collective efficacy through "thinking group." The more commonly taken individual-level perspective can be supplemented by actively considering group-level factors and by working more often with people in groups. Forming and facilitating planning groups consisting of representative members of the target population can provide one concrete way that "thinking group" can be operationalized. Delivering group-based prevention interventions, such as psychoeducation groups, affords another important strategy through which collective efficacy can be activated.

   K. How is use of *Support Systems* (friends, groups, families, communities, organizations, mentors . . .) evidenced?

Social and instrumental support are key components in maintaining positive mental health. Social support is emotionally based, centered on sensitivity, connecting, and caring, such as listening to another's problems. Instrumental support is task related and involves providing tangible assistance when someone needs it, such as helping to change a flat tire. Sometimes both kinds of support occur, such as providing disaster mental health services in a Red Cross shelter, where the volunteer listens and assists with problem solving and also may sweep the floors in an effort to model keeping the shelter clean. Our focus in this discussion is on social support.

Social support can occur naturally, springing from the daily interactions of people in families, communities, and work settings. It also can result through groups that are formed to assist members with managing life events. Support groups and self-help groups are one of the major means through which preventive, promotive, or protective assistance is received (Bloom, 1996). Whether naturally emerging or constructed, social support is associated with healthiness and with reducing isolation, serving to buffer the slings and arrows of daily life.

Assessing the presence and role of social support in a target population and incorporating its principles is mandatory for preventive programming. Questions to ask include: To what degree is social support present? How does it occur? How do people access it? How do they use it? What are its effects? Is more, or less, needed? Of what kind? How might it be introduced?

How could support systems and their use be enhanced?

Thinking of the ecology of prevention (Chronister, McWhirter, & Kerewsky, 2004; Conyne, 2004; Kelly & Hess, 1987) may help prevention planners to become more sensitive to social support. Indeed, this perspective may aid in giving increased consideration to factors that exist outside of more traditional thinking about providing help dominated, as it is, by remedial, individual, interventionist-based concepts and methods.

The first place to assess social support is in naturally occurring settings. Do members of the target population interact with one another? Do they seem to give and get help? Are there structures, organizations, and processes in the local community through which people interact, such as community centers, neighborhood councils, schools, churches, bowling leagues, and other systems? How do people use these structures? How effective are they in their intended purpose and for the somewhat ancillary purpose of bringing people together, out of which might emerge identifiable social support? Do these naturally occurring settings provide opportunities for prevention programming?

The next place to assess social support is in support and self-help groups that have been organized. Are there any in the community? What kinds? How do they work? How many people participate? How effective do they seem to be? Does a need exist to create more or different kinds of these groups? Is there an opportunity for prevention programming in this arena?

System Strengths

An ecological perspective, mentioned above, assumes greater importance as consideration proceeds beyond the individual level and when a more comprehensive analysis of the problem is sought. One aspect of an ecological perspective is to assess how increasingly larger levels of system contribute to and are affected by the problem. Bronfenbrenner (1979) termed these levels the microsystem, mesosystem, exosystem, and macrosystem. The World Health Organization's (WHO, 2004) paper on preventing violence labeled these levels as individual, relationship, community, and societal.

In this complex world it is important that people are ecologically competent (Conyne & Cook, 2004), a concept adapted from Steele's (1973) notion of environmental competence. To be ecologically competent means that persons are capable of negotiating successfully and ethically with their environment. They are concerned not only with happiness, but with well-being in relation to economic cost and impact (New Economic Foundation, 2006; Thompson, 2008).

L. How is *Ecological Competence* evidenced?

Ecologically competent people can do simple things, like cross a busy street. They can find their way to new locations. They are able to perform increasingly more complex tasks, as well. They can find social support when needed. They can influence aspects of their environment. They can relate well with others who are both similar and different from them. They contribute productively and compassionately.

They are good citizens who are sensitive to their environment and those around them. They can anticipate and plan for events. They can resiliently manage crises. They can take advantage of resources without hurting others. They can find or develop strategies for safety and security. They can advocate for necessary change. They are oriented toward such values as interdependence, cooperation, partnerships, and conservation (Capra, 1996).

In terms of interpersonal violence on college campuses, an ecological analysis suggests that all levels of the college system be examined. What aspects are associated with the individual level (e.g., behavior, personality, alcohol/substance abuse, culture, gender), the relationship level (e.g., possible connections between those involved), the community level (e.g., the role played by existing policies, present services), and the societal level (e.g., cultural norms and related practices that may support violence)?

(1) *How ecologically competent are population members?*

The sample characteristics mentioned above that can be associated with ecological competence need to be assessed during problem formulation and throughout program development and delivery. To what degree are these characteristics present in the target population? How are they employed? How ecologically competent are individuals and the target community at large? How could these competencies be incorporated within a campus interpersonal violence prevention program?

(2) *What can population members do and/or what can preventive intervention do to increase ecological competence?*

Prevention planners are encouraged to continually broaden their perspective about human behavior, environmental influence, and the prevention of problems such as interpersonal violence on college campuses. The WHO report on violence prevention, referred to earlier, strongly suggests that a public-health, ecological perspective be adopted for preventing this and other problems. By adopting this perspective, which incorporates attention to issues of cultural relevance and many other factors, ecological competence can be strengthened.

M. How is *Advocacy* evidenced?

Advocacy means to argue in favor of an idea, a cause, or a policy on one's own behalf, in support of others, or of an organization being represented. Advocacy has become an important function for many mental health practitioners, and especially for those conducting prevention, because the sources of numerous problems affecting large numbers of people often can be located within social, political, economic, educational, and health systems (Lewis, Arnold, House, & Toporek, 2002). In many cases, then, a necessary strategy to effect change and to prevent the occurrence of future adversity is to advocate for system change. Advocacy is especially pertinent to support people, organizations, or groups that are powerless or marginalized (Watson, Collins, & Collins Correia, 2004). People can learn advocacy skills by becoming empowered to gain increased power and control without interfering with the rights of others (E. McWhirter, 1994). Or advocates can act on their behalf, asserting their issues to seek a more hospitable system.

> *What can population members do and/or what can preventive intervention do to foster advocacy?*

Considering advocacy in relation to campus interpersonal violence, it may be important to assess the degree to which this issue is being addressed. After all, violence against others is not something that many systems wish to make obvious. It's certainly not good business. Yet in order for focused and constructive progress to be made in identifying the incidence of interpersonal violence, and then in developing prevention programs to lower it, some degree of public attention needs to emerge along with a commitment to action. Advocacy with administration might be necessary to help the institution in its readiness to confront this issue. As well, steps may be taken for advocating on behalf of individuals who have been victimized by interpersonal violence and/or to assist them in determining what course of action they might want to pursue themselves. Finally, prevention programs can be constructed to include advocacy training—of students and of staff—to help foster a safer and more secure academic and living environment.

N. *Summation and Integration:* Based on your above assessment, what factors should be reduced and which ones increased to effect positive preventive activity?

By now a considerable amount of information has been produced from your team's analysis. The planning goal is to lower the stressors contained in the numerator while raising the supports found in the denominator. The overall goal is to apply the prevention program that results from planning to reduce the number of existing cases of interpersonal violence on campus or—better yet, in terms of incidence reduction—*to stop new cases or to slow their rate of increase.*

LEARNING EXERCISE 9.2

Process Check #4

Yes, it is time for another process check. These checks of "how you are doing" are vitally important for effective progress and member satisfaction. So, review your work up to now using the same kinds of process questions as before, and jot a summary statement next:

_____

_____

_____

(Continued)

(Continued)

Sometimes process checks take some courage to conduct, because people tend to be reluctant to expose themselves to feedback. Hey! It could be negative, after all. But that is the very point. It is far better to learn of both positive and negative information along the way, when there is an opportunity to correct it—or to enhance what is working—than at the end, or not at all. Resulting feedback can keep a group on task, help the work to be enjoyable and meaningful, and contribute to good products.

Yet team members need to be open to this kind of interaction, and engaging in process checks needs to become part of the team culture. So, all team members need to ask themselves (and share appropriately with other members):

- How ready am I to give and get feedback?
- Do I know how to do this appropriately and effectively?
- Can I be counted on?

Summary

Correct and concrete problem identification is a key to effective program development. When prevention is the goal, problem identification takes on a unique form because prevention is concerned with stopping or reducing the onset of new cases of a problem or set of problems. We have learned that this approach is called incidence reduction.

This chapter focused on incidence reduction in prevention program development and evaluation by detailing the adapted incidence reduction formula and applying it in a general way to the example we have been following of campus interpersonal violence prevention.

Program development seeks to create conditions where deficit factors (Physical × Social × Culture) contained in the formula's numerator can be reduced. Concomitantly, in the formula's denominator, program development is geared toward increasing strength factors (Personal × Interpersonal × Group × System). Combining the strategy of reducing defects while increasing strengths, when applied in a coherent program development model, can help reach preventive goals centered around lowered numbers of new cases, increasing strengths in participants, and lessening environmental stressors. You will get some practice in applying this approach in the next and final chapter.

CHAPTER 10

Analyzing and Learning From Prevention Programs

Purposes of This Final Chapter

The purposes of this final chapter are to give practical attention to innovative programs in campus interpersonal violence prevention (that have yet to demonstrate empirical support) and to give you opportunities to analyze prevention programs for their inclusion of important prevention components. As I have found through years of teaching prevention, students have found that analyzing prevention programs directly enhances their own learning and their capacity to develop and evaluate prevention programs.

As you will see, the adapted incidence reduction formula can be used to analyze programs. In fact, in addition to being very effective for defining a prevention problem—which is how we have employed it earlier—the formula also proves to be helpful in analyzing existing programs and in designing the contents of new prevention programs. In what follows we will use it to analyze three evolving campus interpersonal violence prevention programs after first getting some experience in examining a prevention program that previously has been judged by experts to be excellent.

Evidence-Based Prevention Programs Are Lacking at College and University Level

Prevention programs in general are concentrated at the early years of development and in schools and families. For instance, by my tally none of the 29 "model" and "promising" evidence-based prevention programs contained in the Blueprints for Violence Prevention database (Center for the Study and Prevention of Violence, 2002–2004) and only 1 of 121 model and promising programs identified by the Substance Abuse and Mental Health Services Administration (SAMHSA) and its National Registry of Effective Prevention Programs (NREPP) are drawn from higher education settings. That prevention programs are concentrated during early development and in schools and families is sensible, given that the largest and longest potential preventive effects can occur with children and adolescents and that they are readily reachable in school and family settings.

However, prevention is important at all age levels and in all settings, and there are many interesting, innovative, and useful programs available. In some cases, evidence-based programs have been documented across the life span (Price, Cowen, Lorion, & Ramos-McKay, 1988). Yet the college and university setting remains largely uncharted, including campus prevention programs in interpersonal violence. Therefore, a virtual "growth industry" exists for prevention researchers to test college and university prevention programs, as well as those intended to prevent campus interpersonal violence, for empirical effectiveness. Although it is highly desirable that prevention programs are validated empirically, valuable programs exist for use that have yet to attain this status, for a number of legitimate reasons. We can still draw, with caution, from those unvalidated programs. As well, researchers need to press forward to the next level, seeking to produce empirical evidence of effectiveness.

Before moving to this discussion of campus-based interpersonal violence prevention programs, though, it will be instructive to examine a prevention program that is considered to be a model. For this purpose, let us examine a program from the Blueprints for Violence Prevention resource bank, the Midwestern Prevention Project (Pentz, Mihalic, & Grotpeter, 1998). Focusing on this program will provide a useful framework that can be utilized when considering the three college-level interpersonal violence programs to follow.

Examining a Model Prevention Program:
The Midwestern Prevention Project

Basic Description

The Midwestern Prevention Project (MPP) is aimed at preventing adolescent drug abuse. It is a comprehensive, community-based, multifaceted approach offered over an extended time period. The program is delivered in schools and also in family and community settings.

This program seeks to reduce environmental stressors expressed through the strong social pressures upon many adolescents to experiment with and use drugs and to increase their skills in avoiding drug use and drug use settings. Program components are organized through a coordinated system of community-level strategies, including (a) mass media programming; (b) a school program with booster sessions, which is the central aspect of this comprehensive approach; (c) a parent education and organization program; and (d) local policy change with reference to alcohol, tobacco, and other drugs.

The MPP follows a Person × Situation × Environment theoretical perspective aimed at reducing incidence, prevalence, and intensity duration. Person-level variables include attention to prior drug use, intention to use, prior skills, prior appraisal, prior social support seeking, and physiological reactions. Training teaches students about peer and social pressures, as well as decision-making skills to resist peer pressures. Situation-level variables include peer influences, prior skills practice with peers, family influences, social support, transitions being experienced, and exposure to drugs. Training focuses on interpersonal, group, and support mechanisms to reduce peer pressure and to increase positive communication. Environmental-level variables include media influences, availability of prevention resources, prevailing community norms, demographic factors, fiscal resources, and school/community policy. Mass media, community organization, and policy change strategies are used to modify sources of environmental stressors.

MPP personnel report the program has produced in participants net reductions of up to 40% in daily smoking and marijuana use, with smaller declines in alcohol use. These gains have been sustained up to Grade 12. In addition, positive outcomes have been realized with parents, where alcohol and marijuana use have declined while constructive parent–child communications about drug use have increased. Policy changes have included institutionalization of the school program and vendor cooperation in refusing to sell tobacco and alcohol to minors. These accomplishments have cost $175,000 over 3 years for all aspects of the program.

Brief Program Analysis

Several criteria appropriate for prevention program analysis were discussed in Chapter 3. You may benefit from referring to those at this point. We will proceed by drawing from aspects of the prevention program development and evaluation approach, with particular attention to the adapted incidence reduction formula.

In order to produce a comprehensive, community-based, multimethod prevention program persisting over several years, such as the MPP, it is likely that planners participated in many—if not all—of the preparatory steps outlined in the prevention program development and evaluation approach: (a) Establish and maintain a team, (b) Identify a potential community issue, (c) Explore related professional literature, (d) Develop a germinal, motivating idea, (e) Engage stakeholder planning council, (f) Create a shared vision and mission, (g) Stimulate community readiness, and (h) Assess. These process steps are community based and build collaboration and cultural relevance while guiding the evolution of sound program ideas.

As they designed the program, the planners also needed to attend to identifying the problem, determining objectives, and selecting strategies, and they plotted activities, tasks, resources, and timelines for these strategies. They created and maintained an evaluation design that encompassed process and outcome variables.

The program description of the MPP does not permit examination of all the above steps, but they are the heart and soul of program development in prevention. What it does do is to allow for examination of the program content, for which the adapted incidence reduction formula, reprinted next, can be used in analysis.

Decrease:	DEFICITS
	Environmental Risks and Stressors: (Physical × Social × Culture)
	Physical Environment: Stressors in Natural and Built Environment
	Social Environment: Stressors in Informal and Formal Social Relations
	Culture: Exploitation, Oppression, Underlying Values and Patterns
Increase:	STRENGTHS
	Protective Factors: (Personal × Interpersonal × Groups × System)
	Personal Factors: Self-Esteem, Well-Being, Resilience, Self-Efficacy
	Interpersonal Factors: Interpersonal and Coping Skills, Engagement
	Group Factors: Collective Efficacy, Social Support
	System Factors: Ecological Competence, Advocacy

The MPP's theoretical emphasis on Person × Situation × Environment is consistent with the adapted incidence reduction formula.

General defect-reduction approaches. Reduction of deficits occurs by using mass media, community organization, and policy change strategies to lessen the effects of peer pressure on drug use and to positively modify the culture surrounding drug use. A parent–principal committee functions to review school drug policy and parent–child communication training.

General strength-increasing approaches. At the same time, skill building and group and social support strategies are used to develop new skills in students and parents alike, as well as to buttress existing strengths. Particular attention is given to building drug resistance skills, to setting avoidance strategies, and to learning more adaptive ways for students and their parents to communicate about drugs and other matters.

LEARNING EXERCISE 10.1

Assessing Your Understanding of the Prevention Program Development and Evaluation Approach

Applying the adapted incidence reduction formula to a model prevention program (the MPP) provided you with an opportunity to examine a good program. Doing so can yield insights about how to create good programs yourself.

At this point, how confident are you feeling about the prevention program development and evaluation approach?

- Circle below how adequately you understand the approach:

Fully	Mostly	Somewhat	Slightly

If you answered "somewhat" or "slightly," how might your understanding be improved?

_____

_____

_____

_____

- To what extent do you think you might be able to use the approach, or at least parts of it?

_____

_____

_____

Turning to Campus Interpersonal Violence Prevention

The American College Health Association (ACHA) identified national health objectives in its document *Healthy Campus 2010* (ACHA, 2002). These objectives are intended to provide guidance for college health programs leading to improved student health. A key campus health indicator identified in these objectives revolves around injury and violence prevention. Specifically, the ACHA targets reductions in:

Homicides

Physical assaults

Intimate partner violence

Campus dating violence

Racial, ethnic, and gender-based violence, and homophobic intimidation

Emotional abuse

Sexual assault

Stalking

Hazing

Suicide, homicide

Aggravated assault

Attacks on faculty and staff

Rape and attempted rape

Physical fighting

Weapon carrying (Carr, 2005)

I listed these forms of campus violence in a column to emphasize the numerous ways it occurs. Indeed, between 1995 and 2002 some 479,000 crimes of campus violence occurred annually, with these reported numbers probably falling well below the actual numbers due to underreporting. Here is but a sampling (Baum & Klaus, 2005):

Approximately 15%–20% of female college students have experienced forced intercourse.

Rape/sexual assault was the only violent crime against students more likely to be committed by someone they knew.

Alcohol and drugs were implicated in some 55%–74% of campus sexual assaults.

20% of faculty, staff, and students surveyed were fearful of their personal safety due to their sexual orientation or gender.

36% of lesbian, gay, bisexual, and transgender (LGBT) students experienced harassment during the past year.

What factors may lead to such figures? Kilmartin (2001) pointed to destructive aspects of a masculine-oriented environment, featuring a continuum of disrespect toward women. Such a perspective reflects a general culture of racism, sexism, and homophobia that influences how some students may view gender, ethnicity, race, sexual identity, and interpersonal relationships.

Many minority students have reported that the college culture they encounter in predominately white campuses can be hostile to them. Such an oppressive culture can lead to intimidation, harassment, and eventually to hate crimes, just because someone is "different."

A major factor in relational violence on campuses is traced to abuse of alcohol and other drugs. For instance, 71% of reported forced sexual touching and 79% of unwanted sexual intercourse occurred under the influence of alcohol (Presley, Meilman, & Cashin, 1997).

First-year students generally are at special risk for victimization. They are new to campus and perhaps less developed than others in having formed boundaries and self-protection strategies. They also are often placed in high-density living situations where interpersonal experimentation is occurring.

In view of these and other factors associated with campus interpersonal violence, the ACHA presented a position statement that is clear in its view of how oppression and injustice are injurious to human rights and contribute to violence and bias:

> We, the members of the Association, believe that for a campus community to be truly healthy, it must be guided by the values of multicultural inclusion, respect, and equality. Intolerance has no place at an institution of higher learning. The Association supports all individuals regardless of sexual orientation, race, national origin, age, religion, or disability. We encourage campus health professionals to be actively engaged in the struggle to end oppression, to prevent bias-related violence in our campus communities, and to take action to eradicate injustice. (Carr, 2005, p. 1)

LEARNING EXERCISE 10.2

Planning a Prevention Program to Reduce Interpersonal Violence

I'd like you now to shift gears from your own prevention topic to consider the information presented in this section's introduction that was drawn from ACHA sources and addresses interpersonal violence on college campuses. Think, also, of the prevention program development and evaluation approach that you've been reading about throughout this book.

In general, how might you go about developing a prevention program to address interpersonal violence occurrences on a campus? You might want to use a separate piece of paper to map out your thinking. Here are some hints:

- Consider the concept of incidence reduction: How does it apply?
- Plan how you might go about "laying the groundwork" (see Steps 1–8 of the prevention program development and evaluation approach) for prevention: What steps might you take?
- Identify what factors you might want to reduce or to increase. Refer to the adapted incidence reduction factors for guidance.

Take 30 minutes to plan your approach. Sketch out your responses to the three areas above. What do you find? Please do not proceed in reading until you have followed these steps.

What Might Be Done?

With an incidence reduction approach that emphasizes community, cultural relevance, and collaboration—the approach we are working with here—we are interested in trying to lessen the number of *new* cases, or the *rate of development* of new cases of interpersonal violence. We would want to develop a collaborative planning team, including representatives of the campus community and to be sure to be sensitive to the campus culture and to population subgroups. We would move through team formation, using group processes to develop and share baseline information about the extent of the problem, develop some possible ideas about how to address it preventively by referring to evidence-based programs that are pertinent, and then to seek broader campus support as we move ahead. We then might expand our planning team and begin to specify more clearly aspects of the problem from an incidence reduction perspective. We would identify what factors contribute to the problem at hand and think about strategies to reduce the intensity of those environmental factors. At the same time we would seek to identify strength factors in our targeted population. The general directions that emerge would then be detailed into concrete plans: who is responsible for the program, what will be done, by whom, when, and with what resources. These specific plans would be set within an evaluation design that would evolve process information, that would assist with guiding and shaping the program, and with outcome information, that would help to determine if new cases of campus interpersonal violence were lowered by the program and if the campus environment and student resources were enhanced beyond what they were prior to the program.

A prevention program aimed at lessening new cases of interpersonal violence on campus would give specific attention to the culture of the campus. What are the risk factors that serve to increase interpersonal violence, such as hazing, binge drinking, intolerance for individual and cultural differences, unsafe parts of campus, ambiguous student code of conduct policy, offices that typically work independently, and unclear expectations for what is acceptable behavior on campus? What are the strengths that students possess and how can they be enhanced? Can male students be enlisted to more obviously support females, might problem-solving and interpersonal skill training be made available, could support groups be established to address issues related to interpersonal violence, and so on?

Analyze Three Program Examples of College Interpersonal Violence Prevention

Many evidence-based prevention programs exist today, as you have read, and easily accessible sources exist for discovering them (see Chapter 3, and Conyne, 2004). However, consistent with my observation at the start of this chapter that, in general, reports of evidence-based prevention programs on college and university campuses are lacking, no descriptions seem to exist in the area of interpersonal violence prevention on college campuses. This may be the case because interpersonal violence largely is a hidden epidemic; these programs are relatively new, and being able to produce and measure preventive effects during the short life of a college generation poses a significant challenge. So this is a growth area for prevention programming and evaluation just waiting for you and others to address.

However, interesting and innovative programs have been launched. What follows is a brief review of some of these programs. Following each one, you will be given an opportunity to apply what you have been reading by analyzing program components using the adapted incidence reduction formula.

Program A: Preventing Violence Against Women Through a Consortium

Colleges and universities are generally safe environments. However, they are not "safe havens," as violent crimes of various kinds occur on all campuses. One particular pernicious strain of such crimes encompasses violence against women. Stalking, domestic violence, and sexual assault typify these crimes.

Women experience considerably more relationship violence and suffer more chronic and injurious assaults than do men. For instance, about one quarter of women report being raped or physically assaulted during their lives by a current or former spouse, date, or cohabiting partner (National Institute of Justice & Centers for Disease Control, 2000). This compares with 7.6% of men who report being victims of similar violence.

Emotional abuse may occur simultaneously with physical abuse and is a predictor for victimization. The frequency of acts of sexual violence against women on college campuses is startling. One of five young women on campus report being forced to have sexual intercourse (Division of Adolescent and School Health, 1995).

Jamestown College (Pranke, 2006) leads a consortium of six North Dakota campuses in combating such violence against women. This consortium, known as ND WEAV (North Dakotans Working in Education Against Violence), is working in cooperation with the North Dakota Council on Abused Women's Services (NDCAWS). The consortium, comprising higher education institutions, community service organizations, and a state government agency, interlaces policy, education, and social support in its prevention effort. With funding from the Justice Department's Violence Against Women Office, the consortium's intent is to make the six participating campuses safe for all women while attending in a focused way to traditionally underserved populations, such as Native American women.

Major strategies being pursued by the Consortium are to:

Reduce Campus Disorganization. Each campus involved in the consortium has constructed a coordinated community response that features a campus advisory committee. The advisory committee consists of representatives from campus administration, faculty, students, staff, security, law enforcement, a domestic violence agency, and victims. The campus advisory committee is charged with developing a coordinated community response to prevent violence against campus women, respond to it effectively when it occurs, and hold perpetrators accountable for their actions. The ultimate goal of the campus advisory committee is to promote an environment that reduces crime against women and provides an optimal response to victims when crime does occur.

Increase Knowledge and Education. Broad-based education is used to reach virtually every person on campus so they can become aware of efforts to prevent and respond to crimes of violence. A primary objective is to improve each student's understanding of violence against women as it relates to campus issues. Key people receive specific information. All incoming students participate in mandatory education regarding prevention of violence against women. Campus security and police gain expertise in order to respond more effectively to sexual assault, domestic violence, and stalking.

A majority of this education occurs during the College, Character, and Career classes required of incoming students. Faculty, staff, campus disciplinary boards, and the student body at large also participate.

Increase Service to Victims Through Advocacy. A victim advocate was hired to oversee the improvement of services for victims of violence and to coordinate the range of educational activities being delivered. Some of the services provided by the advocate are:

- Working to provide emergency response and support for campus women who are victims of violence
- Leading and coordinating activities of the campus advisory committee
- Working to improve campus policies concerning violence against women on campus
- Encouraging and enhancing the ability of the victim to continue with her education by working with academic, housing, and work-study personnel as well as with local police and campus security
- Forming and leading support groups
- Coordinating multidisciplinary training and providing outreach to specific campus populations (e.g., cultural groups, student government, religious organizations)
- Increasing the awareness level of the campus community on issues relating to violence against women on campus
- Gathering information to track the incidence and effect of violence against women on campus
- Working with peer educators to serve as models for helping and to assist with campus education

Analyze Program A: Use the adapted incidence reduction formula to analyze the program. What deficit-reduction strategies may be used? What strength-increasing ones? How might they be evaluated? What did you learn as you analyzed this program?

Write a summary paragraph about each area below:

Deficit-reduction strategies used:

_____

_____

_____

Strength-increasing strategies used:

_____

_____

_____

What evaluation strategies might you suggest?

_____

_____

_____

What did you learn from analyzing this program?

_____

_____

_____

Program B: Sexual Assault Prevention
Through an Online Campus Course Module

The Sexual Assault Prevention and Counseling (SAPAC) office at the University of Nevada–Reno was established in 1996 to reduce the incidence of sexual assault on its campus (SAPAC, n.d.). The SAPAC offers sexual assault prevention programs for male, female, and mixed-gender populations; free and confidential psychotherapy to those who have been assaulted; and academic liaison services for students whose lives have been disrupted because of the assault. These programs consist of classroom presentations by the program coordinator or by trained peer educators (students) who are knowledgeable in the topic. A unique offering consists of an online learning module that is part of a Psychology 101 course.

This online module contains information about prevention, sexual assault, and treatment approaches for sexual assault. A series of slides present myths and beliefs about sexual assault, asking students to answer true or false, followed by the correct answer and explanatory information. All of the slides contain a photo or picture, and some include sound. A quiz worth 20 points to the final course grade concludes the module.

Here is one example that I've drawn from a slide (#17; SAPAC, n.d., http://www.scs.unr.edu/~sapac/101/24verbal.html) that addresses an erroneous belief about sexual assualt: Sexual assault involves only physical, not verbal, coercion. First, the false belief is presented and viewers are quizzed if they think it is true or false. Then, a photograph is presented of a male and female couple with the female in the foreground appearing to be concerned. An accompanying audio track contains the male partner's voice containing a verbally coercive message threatening that no sex means no continued relationship and that he will spread vicious rumors about the female partner unless she complies. The learning episode concludes with presentation of a fact to counteract the preceding myth: Threats, tone of voice, or strong insistence from the male for sex can lead the woman feel as if she has to submit to sexual activity.

This online module focuses on increasing students' knowledge of prevention, sexual assault, and treatment options. Therefore, it is located securely in the denominator, the strengths-based component of the incidence reduction equation. As a required portion of a course that is required for all undergraduate students, it represents a form of universal prevention, cast across the entire campus student population. Its creative use of information technology and the ability to complete the course module at one's own speed would seem to be attractive to many students. Conversely, prevention programs that rely solely on provision of information have a poor track record in changing behavior or in sustaining behavior change. This program seems cognizant of that reality, as it provides referral possibilities within the program and, of course, the online module is one of several other prevention programs offered by the SAPAC office.

Analyze Program B: Use the adapted incidence reduction formula to analyze the program. What deficit-reduction strategies may be used? What strength-increasing ones? How might they be evaluated? What did you learn as you analyzed this program?

Write a summary paragraph about each area below:

Deficit-reduction strategies used:

_____

_____

_____

Strength-increasing strategies used:

_____

_____

_____

What evaluation strategies might you suggest?

_____

_____

_____

What did you learn from analyzing this program?

_____

_____

_____

Program C: Using Theater and Other Strategies to Reduce Interpersonal Violence

Voices Against Violence (referred to earlier in this book) is a comprehensive prevention program at the University of Texas at Austin (Meyers, 2008), whose centerpiece is the use of theater. It was founded in 2000 after receiving a grant from the Department of Justice's Office of Violence Against Women. The result of a collaborative effort involving police from the university and the city of Austin, faculty, students, and on- and off-campus housing personnel, the program's focus is to combat relationship violence, sexual assault, and stalking on college campuses.

The program provides training, outreach, and advocacy instruction. Because the primary strategies aim to increase awareness, knowledge, and skills, they fall within the denominator, the strengths-based component of the adapted incidence reduction formula. However, note that by providing these skill-based experiences, the program also influences the capacity of the environment to become more responsive and supportive. For example, campus security and police receive specific training to bolster their abilities to interact sensitively and effectively with victims and first responders, which, by extension, reduces a potential source of environmental threat. The advocacy function also impinges on the environment, helping survivors of sexual assault to obtain safer housing, identifying legal assistance from within the community, and drawing from a small emergency fund that can provide basic assistance. Awareness of sexual assault prevention is increased through special events (e.g., "Take Back the Night"), information tables, and video presentations.

The Voices Against Violence peer theater group is its most recognizable component. Based on principles of the Theater of the Oppressed (Boal, 2000), performances about sexual abuse are tailored to targeted audiences and seek to stimulate dialogue between the performers and audience members. The 16 student actors learn about sexual assault issues through a special two-semester class and then adapt scenarios about relationship dynamics into performances that fit the culture and experience of any specific audience.

Anecdotal evidence only is available. Reports have been received that students seem more able to identify and control behavior related to interpersonal violence, and the number of students coming for counseling about relationship violence is increasing.

Analyze Program C: Use the adapted incidence reduction formula to analyze the program. What deficit-reduction strategies may be used? What strength-increasing ones? How might they be evaluated? What did you learn as you analyzed this program? Finally, as this program is the last one you will analyze, take a summative view of your learning by responding to this question: In sum, what did you learn about prevention program development and evaluation by analyzing these three programs?

Write a summary paragraph about each area below:

Deficit-reduction strategies used:

_____

_____

_____

Strength-increasing strategies used:

_____

_____

_____

What evaluation strategies might you suggest?

_____

_____

_____

What did you learn from analyzing this program?

_____

_____

_____

In sum, what did you learn about prevention program development and evaluation by analyzing all three programs?

_____

_____

_____

Summary

This final chapter provided opportunities to practice analyzing three emerging programs in the area of campus interpersonal violence prevention. This experience is intended to help you integrate and apply what you have been learning in your reading and study of prevention program development and evaluation.

The observation was made in the chapter that few empirically based programs in higher education have been identified. This dearth of material represents a vital area for future research and development in prevention.

Leading up to analysis of the three campus interpersonal violence programs (ND WEAV, a consortium; SAPAC, an online course module; Voices Against Violence, featuring a theater approach), an empirically validated prevention program listed in the Blueprints for Violence Prevention resource bank, the Midwestern Prevention Project (Pentz et al., 1998), was described and analyzed briefly using the adapted incidence reduction formula.

Gaining experience reading, reviewing, and analyzing innovative and effective prevention programs by using accepted criteria for success can enhance program development skills in prevention. That is, after all, the main purpose of this book: that you will become more adept at understanding prevention program development and evaluation and then be able to do it well.

I wish you the very best as you move ahead in the area of prevention. Bidding farewell, I will leave you on a light note with a valuable everyday prevention practice, indeed, one that has found its way into many effective prevention programs—the social support that can be found through reaching out.

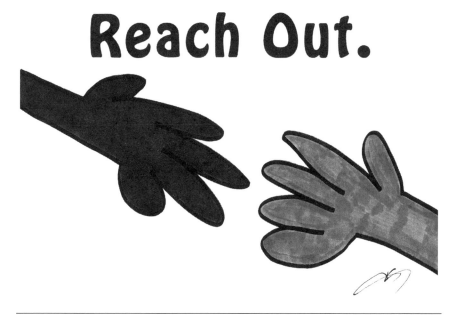

Figure 10.1   Social Support Through Reaching Out

Source: © John Conyne.

Appendix A

Ten-Step PPD&E Model

A. LAY THE GROUNDWORK (Steps 1–8) for Community, Collaboration and Cultural Relevance
STEP 1: Establish and maintain a team
STEP 2: Identify a potential community issue
STEP 3: Explore related professional literature
STEP 4: Develop a germinal, motivating idea
STEP 5: Engage stakeholder planning council
STEP 6: Create a shared vision and mission
STEP 7: Stimulate community readiness

STEP 8: Assess
    a. Conduct a local ecological assessment
    b. Search for evidence-based programs

B. IMPLEMENT AND EVALUATE (Steps 9–10)
STEP 9: Design the prevention program plan
STEP 10: Design the prevention program evaluation plan

Appendix B

*Laying the Groundwork
(Steps 1–8) for Community,
Collaboration, and Cultural Relevance*

STEP 1: Establish and maintain a team

STEP 2: Identify a potential community issue

STEP 3: Explore related professional literature

STEP 4: Develop a germinal, motivating idea

STEP 5: Engage stakeholder planning council

STEP 6: Create a shared vision and mission

STEP 7: Stimulate community readiness

STEP 8: Assess
   a. Conduct local ecological assessment
   b. Search for evidence-based programs

Appendix C

Implement and Evaluate (Steps 9–10)

STEP 9:   Design the prevention program plan
STEP 10: Design the prevention program evaluation plan

Appendix D

PPD&E Step 9: Design the Prevention Program Plan

a. Determine problem in general terms

b. Use adapted incidence reduction formula

c. Set objectives

d. Choose among alternative strategies

e. Plan implementation

- Objective
- Strategies
- Activities
- Tasks
- Resources
- Timelines

Appendix E

PPD&E Step 10

Design the Prevention Program Evaluation Plan

---

a. Process/formative evaluation

Key prevention processes:

- Context considered
- Community orientation
- Cultural relevance/fit
- Collaboration/partnerships
- Fidelity
- Guided adaptability
- Evidence based

---

b. Outcome/summative evaluation

Key prevention questions:

- Were new cases eliminated or diminished?
- Were deficits reduced?
- Was the environment improved?
- Were strengths and natural supports increased?

Key prevention criteria:

- Adequacy, appropriateness
- Effectiveness, efficiency
- Side effects, sustainability
- Transferability, dissemination
- Usefulness and general contribution

Appendix F

Basic Incidence
Reduction Formulae

A. Original Albee Incidence Reduction Formula

Decrease: $$\frac{(\text{Organic Factors} + \text{Stress} + \text{Exploitation})}{(\text{Self-Esteem} + \text{Coping Skills} + \text{Support Groups})}$$
Increase:

B. Adapted Incidence Reduction Formula: GENERAL Version

Decrease: DEFICITS

$$\frac{\text{Environmental Risks and Stressors: (Physical} \times \text{Social} \times \text{Culture)}}{\text{Protective Factors: (Personal} \times \text{Interpersonal} \times \text{Group} \times \text{System)}}$$

Increase: STRENGTHS

C. Adapted Incidence Reduction Formula: PLANNING Version

Decrease: DEFICITS

Environmental Risks and Stressors: (Physical × Social × Culture)
Physical Environment: Stressors in Natural and Built Environment
Social Environment: Stressors in Informal and Formal Social Relations
Culture: Exploitation, Oppression, Underlying Values and Patterns

Increase: STRENGTHS

Protective Factors: (Personal × Interpersonal × Groups × System)
Personal Factors: Self-Esteem, Well-Being, Resilience, Self-Efficacy
Interpersonal Factors: Interpersonal and Coping Skills, Engagement
Group Factors: Collective Efficacy, Social Support
System Factors: Ecological Competence, Advocacy

Appendix G

PPD&E Step 9b

Identify the Problem

Adapted Incidence Reduction Formula for Problem Identification in Prevention Program Development and Evaluation

Decrease: DEFICITS

> *Environmental Risks and Stressors: (Physical × Social × Culture)*
> **Physical Environment:** Stressors in Natural and Built Environment
> **Social Environment:** Stressors in Informal and Formal Social Relations
> **Culture:** Exploitation, Oppression, Underlying Values and Patterns

Increase: STRENGTHS

> *Protective Factors: (Personal × Interpersonal × Group × System)*
> **Personal Factors:** Self-Esteem, Well-Being, Resilience, Self-Efficacy
> **Interpersonal Factors:** Interpersonal and Coping Skills, Engagement
> **Group Factors:** Collective Efficacy, Social Support
> **System Factors:** Ecological Competence, Advocacy

I. Contributions to Environmental Deficits (Numerator Factors)

Reduce Environmental Deficits

Physical Environment Stressors

    A.   What *Physical Environmental Stressors* (natural and built environment, context, events, circumstances, situations) affect the lives of people in this population?

(1) *What organic physical, mental, or emotional behaviors are affected by physical environmental stressors? (e.g., Down syndrome, lead poisoning, depression, obesity, attention deficit, alcoholism)*

(2) *How do they inhibit functioning, and what is their strength?*

(3) *What physical stressors are present that could affect any in the population?*

(4) *How could physical stressors be reduced by population members and/or by preventive intervention?*

Social Environment Stressors

B. What *Social Environmental Stressors* exist that can lead to psychological and emotional disorders?

(1) *What could be done by population members and/or by preventive intervention to reduce negative effects of the social environment?*

(2) *How can negative behaviors be reduced?*

Cultural Stressors in the Environment

C. What is there about the environmental *Culture* that may support exploitation and affect the lives of people in this population?

(1) *Identify any abuse: Oppression? Exploitation? Marginalization? Violence?*

(2) *Describe how any oppression and exploitation are expressed in terms of ethnicity, race, gender, sexual orientation, age, religious orientation, spiritual affiliation, socioeconomic status, and physical/mental ability.*

(3) *How could this oppression and exploitation be reduced by population members and/or by preventive intervention?*

II. Contributions to Personal, Interpersonal, Group, and System Strengths (Denominator Factors)

Increase Protective Strengths

Personal Strengths

D. How is *Self-Esteem* evidenced?

(1) *What competencies tend to be shown?*

(2) *What could be done by population members and/or by preventive intervention to enhance self-esteem?*

E. How is *Well-Being* evidenced?

(1) *What competencies tend to be shown?*

(2) *What could be done by population members and/or by preventive intervention to enhance well-being?*

F. How is *Resilience* evidenced?

    (1) *What competencies tend to be shown?*

    (2) *What could be done by population members and/or by preventive intervention to enhance their resilience?*

G. How is *Self-Efficacy* evidenced?

    (1) *What competencies tend to be shown?*

    (2) *What could be done by population members and/or by preventive intervention to enhance their sense of personal self-efficacy?*

Interpersonal Strengths

H. How are *Interpersonal* and *Coping Skills* evidenced?

    (1) *What competencies tend to be shown?*
- Interpersonal skills
- Coping skills

    (2) *What could be done by population members and/or by preventive intervention to enhance their interpersonal skills?*

I. How is *Engagement* evidenced?

    (1) *What competencies tend to be shown?*

    (2) *What could be done by population members and/or by preventive intervention to enhance their ability to become engaged?*

Group Strengths

J. How is *Collective Efficacy* evidenced?

    What could be done by population group members and/or by preventive intervention to enhance their sense of collective efficacy?

K. How is use of *Support Systems* (friends, groups, families, communities, organizations, mentors . . .) evidenced?

    How could support systems and their use be enhanced?

System Strengths

L. How is *Ecological Competence* evidenced?

    (1) *How ecologically competent are population members?*

    (2) *What can population members do and/or what can preventive intervention do to increase ecological competence?*

M. How is *Advocacy* evidenced?

    What can population members do and/or what can preventive intervention do to foster advocacy?

N. *Summation and Integration:* Based on your above assessment, what factors should be reduced and which ones increased to effect positive preventive activity?

Set objectives
Choose among alternative strategies
Planning implementation: • Objective • Strategies • Activities • Tasks • Resources • Timelines
PPD&E Step 10: Design Evaluation
Design process/formative evaluation
Design outcome/summative evaluation
Plan for Sustainability
Plan for Replication and Transferability
Plan for Dissemination and Usefulness

Appendix H

Useful Web Sites

Development Services Group, Inc., is in the process of developing a resource manual for supplemental assistance in obtaining indicator information. These materials will be completed and distributed in the near future. In the meantime, the following online sources contain indicator information:

Behavioral Health Research Center of the Southwest: http://www.bhrcs.org

Blueprints for Violence Prevention, Center for the Study and Prevention of Violence, University of Colorado: http://www.colorado.edu/cspv/blueprints

Bureau of Justice Statistics Web site: http://www.ojp.usdoj.gov/bjs/pubalp2.htm

Center for Adolescent Studies, Indiana University: http://education.indiana.edu/cas/cashmpg.html

Centers for the Application of Prevention Technologies (CAPT), national Web site (contains links to CAPTs by region): http://www.captus.org

Western CAPT: http://www.unr.edu/westcapt

Census Bureau: http://www.census.gov

Centers for Disease Control and Prevention: http://www.cdc.gov

Centers for Disease Control, Youth Risk Behavior System Survey 2003: http://www.cdc.gov/nccdphp/dash/yrbs

Centers for Substance Abuse Prevention (CSAP): http://www.samhsa.gov/csap/index.htm

CSAP's Decision Support System (DSS): http://www.preventiondss.org

Child Trends DataBank: http://www.childtrendsdatabank.org/whatsnew.cfm

Department of Health and Human Services (DHHS), Trends in the Well-Being of America's Children and Youth, 1999: http://aspe.gov/hsp/99trends/index.htm

Drug and Alcohol Treatment and Prevention Global Network: http://www.drugnet.net

Exemplary and Promising Safe, Disciplined and Drug-Free Schools Programs 2001; Safe, Disciplined and Drug-Free Schools Expert Panel, U.S. Department of Education: http://www.ed.gov/admins/lead/safety/exemplary01/exemplary01.pdf

Join Together Online: http://www.jointogether.org

Juvenile Justice Evaluation Center, Justice Research Statistics Association: http://www.jrsa.org/jjec

Kids Count (Annie E. Casey Foundation): http://www.aecf.org/kidscount/kc2000

National Center for Education Statistics: http://nces.ed.gov/http://nces.ed.gov

National Criminal Justice Reference Service: http://www.ncjrs.org

Office of Juvenile Justice and Delinquency Prevention (OJJDP): http://ojjdp.ncjrs.org

OJJDP Model Programs Guide (OJJDP and DSG, Inc.): http://www.dsgonline.com/projects_titlev.html http://www.dsgonline.com/projects_titlev.html http://www.dsgonline.com/mpg_index.htm

OJJDP Strategic Planning Tool: http://www.iir.com/nygc/tool/default.htm

OJJDP's Statistical Briefing Book (SBB): http://ojjdp.ncjrs.org/ojstatbb

Office of National Drug Control Policy (ONDCP) Institute: http://www.WhiteHousedrugpolicy.gov

Preventing Crime: What Works, What Doesn't, What's Promising, A Report to the United States Congress, University of Maryland: http://www.ncjrs.org/works

Prevention Online (PREVLINE): http://www.health.org

SAMHSA Prevention Platform: http://www.preventionplatform.samhsa.gov/macro

Search Institute: http://www.search-institute.org

Strengthening America's Families, Effective Family Programs for Prevention of Delinquency, Department of Health Promotion and Education, University of Utah: http://www.strengtheningfamilies.org

Substance Abuse and Mental Health Services Administration (SAMHSA) Model Programs, U.S. Department of Health and Human Services: http://modelprograms.samhsa.gov/template.cfm?page=default

U.S. Department of Education Nation's Record Card 1998: http://nces.ed.gov/nationsreportcard

U.S. Department of Justice, Federal Bureau of Investigation (FBI), Uniform Crime Reports: http://www.fbi.gov/ucr/ucr.htm

Youth Violence: A Report of the Surgeon General, U. S. Department of Health and Human Services, Centers for Disease Control and Prevention, National Center for Injury Prevention, Substance Abuse and Mental Health Services Administration, Center for Mental Health Services, and National Institutes of Health: http://www .surgeongeneral.gov/library/youthviolence/toc.html

If you or any member of your community team are aware of any Web site addresses (or other sources) that you find helpful and believe should be added to the resource guide, please feel free to contact DSG with your suggestions (call 1–877–5-TITLE-5 [584–8535]).

References

Adams, E. (2008). Moving from contemplation to preparation: Is counseling psychology ready to embrace culturally responsive prevention? *The Counseling Psychologist, 35,* 840–849.

Agency for Healthcare Research and Quality. (2008a). *Put prevention into practice.* Washington, DC: U.S. Department of Health and Human Services. Retrieved March 11, 2008, from http://ahrq.hhs.gov/clinic/ppipix.htm

Agency for Healthcare Research and Quality. (2008b). *Real men wear gowns.* Washington, DC: U.S. Department of Health and Human Services. Retrieved May 20, 2008, from http://www.ahrq.gov/realmen/

Albee, G. (1980). A competency model must replace the defect model. In L. Bond & J. Rosen (Eds.), *Competency and coping during adulthood* (pp. 75–104). Hanover, NH: University Press of New England.

Albee, G. (1982). Preventing psychopathology and promoting human potential. *American Psychologist, 37,* 1043–1050.

Albee, G. (1985). The argument for primary prevention. *Journal of Primary Prevention, 5,* 213–219.

Albee, G. (1986). Toward a just society: Lessons from observations on the primary prevention of psychopathology. *American Psychologist, 41,* 891–898.

Albee, G., & Gullotta, T. (Eds.). (1997). *Primary prevention works.* Thousand Oaks, CA: Sage.

American Academy of Periodontology. (2005). *Mouth-body connection.* Retrieved March 17, 2008, from http://www.perio.org/consumer/mbc.top2.htm

American College Health Association. (2002, September). *Healthy campus 2010: Making it happen.* Baltimore, MD: Author.

American Counseling Association. (2008a). *Advocacy competencies.* Retrieved May 20, 2008, from http://www.counseling.org/Resources/

American Counseling Association. (2008b). *Hawaii fun facts* [ACA '08 annual conference and exposition advance registration brochure]. Alexandria, VA: Author.

American Psychological Association. (2002). Guidelines on multicultural education, training, research, practice, and organization change for psychologists. *American Psychologist, 61,* 271–285. Retrieved June 10, 2008, from http://www.apa.org/pi/multiculturalguidelines.pdf

American Psychological Association. (2003). *Guidelines on multicultural education, training, research, practice, and organizational change for psychologists.* Washington, DC: Author.

American Psychological Association. (2008a). *Organizational purposes* [APA Bylaw 1.1]. Retrieved November 6, 2008, from http://www.apa.org/about

American Psychological Association. (2008b). *Psychologically healthy workplace awards and best practice honors 2008*. Washington, DC: APA Psychologically Healthy Workplace Program. Retrieved November 6, 2008, from www.PHWA.org

American Psychological Association. (2008c, October). *Stress in America*. Retrieved November 3, 2008, from www.nyspa.org

American Psychological Association Commission on Violence and Youth. (1996). *Is youth violence just another fact of life?* Retrieved January 21, 2008, from http://www.apa.org/ppo/issues/pbviolence.html

American Psychological Association Presidential Task Force on Evidence-Based Practice. (2006). Evidenced-based practice in psychology. *American Psychologist, 61,* 271–285.

Anderson, N. (2008). Our duty to an overweight nation. *Monitor on Psychology, 39,* 9.

Arredondo, P., Tovar-Blank, Z., & Parham, T. (2008). Challenges and promises of becoming a culturally competent counselor in a sociopolitical era of change and empowerment. *Journal of Counseling & Development, 86,* 261–268.

Aspinall, L., & Staudinger, U. (Eds.). (2003). *A psychology of human strengths: Fundamental questions and future directions for a positive psychology*. Washington, DC: American Psychological Association.

Association for Specialists in Group Work. (1998). *Principles for diversity-competent group workers*. Retrieved June 11, 2008, from http://www.asgw.org/PDF/Principles_for_Diversity.pdf

Ballard, D. (2008, October 29). *Effective and ethical marketing strategies for psychologists*. Presentation at the annual meeting of the Ohio Psychological Association, Columbus, OH.

Bandura, A. (1997). *Self-efficacy: The exercise of control*. New York: Freeman.

Baum, K., & Klaus, P. (2005, January). *Violent victimization of college students* (NCI Publication No. 206836). Washington, DC: U.S. Department of Justice, Office of Justice Programs, Bureau of Justice Statistics.

Baumeister, R. (1998). The self. In D. Gilbert, S. Fiske, & G. Lindzey (Eds.), *The handbook of social psychology* (pp. 680–740). New York: Random House.

Baumeister, R., Smart, L., & Boden, J. (1996). Relation of threatened egotism to violence and aggression: The dark side of self-esteem. *Psychological Review, 103,* 5–33.

Baye, B. (2008, November 8). Obama's record of listening—yes, as a community organizer—pays off. *Cincinnati Enquirer,* Opinions section, p. D-7.

Belch, J., MacCuish, A., Campbell, I., Taylor, R., Prescott, R., Lee, R., et al. (2008, October 16). The prevention of arterial disease and diabetes (POPADAD) trial: Factorial randomized placebo in patients with diabetes and asymptomatic arterial disease. *BMJ, 337,* a1840. Retrieved October 19, 2008, from http://www.bmj.com/cgi/content/full/337/oct16_2/a1840

Bemak, F., & Chi-Ying Chung, R. (2008). New professional roles and advocacy strategies for school counselors: A multicultural/social justice perspective to move beyond the nice counselor syndrome. *Journal of Counseling & Development, 86,* 372–381.

Biglan, A., Mrazek, P., Carnine, D., & Flay, B. (2003). The integration of research and practice in the prevention of youth problem behaviors. *American Psychologist, 58,* 433–440.

Bloom, M. (1996). *Primary prevention practices*. Thousand Oaks, CA: Sage.

Boal, A. (2000). *Theater of the oppressed*. London: Pluto Press.

Boone, P. (1958). *'Twixt twelve and twenty*. Upper Saddle River, NJ: Prentice Hall.

Botvin, G., Baker, E., Dusenbury, L., Botvin, E., & Diaz, T. (1995). Long-term follow-up results of a randomized drug abuse prevention trial in a white middle-class population. *Journal of the American Medical Association, 14,* 1106–1112.

Botvin, G., & Tortu, S. (1988). Preventing adolescent substance abuse through life skills training. In R. Price, E. Cowen, R. Lorion, & J. Ramos-McKay (Eds.), *14 ounces of prevention: A casebook for practitioners* (pp. 98–110). Washington, DC: American Psychological Association.

Brand, E., Lakey, B., & Berman, S. (1995). A preventive, psychoeducational approach to increase perceived social support. *American Journal of Community Psychology, 23,* 117–135.

Branden, N. (1994). *The six pillars of self-esteem.* New York: Bantam Books.

Brim, O., Ryff, C., & Kessler, R. (Eds.). (2004). *How healthy are we? A national study of well-being at midlife.* Chicago: University of Chicago Press.

Bronfenbrenner, U. (1979). *The ecology of human development.* Cambridge, MA: Harvard University Press.

Brown, N. (2008). *Curriculum for psychoeducational groups.* New York: American Group Psychotherapy Association.

Bruvold, W. (1993). A meta-analysis of adolescent smoking prevention programs. *American Journal of Public Health, 83,* 6872–6880.

Bruzzese, A. (2008, April 16). Health on the job: Watch for warnings of alcoholism. *Cincinnati Enquirer,* p. E-2.

Buettner, D. (2008a). *The blue zone: Lessons for living longer from the people who've lived the longest.* Washington, DC: National Geographic Society.

Buettner, D. (2008b, May-June). Living health to 100. *AARP the Magazine,* 67–69, 91.

Byrd, T., & Reininger, B. (2009). Promoting health lifestyles. In M. Kenny, A. Horne, P. Orpinas, & L. Reese (Eds.), *Realizing social justice: The challenge of preventive interventions* (pp. 250–278). Washington, DC: American Psychological Association.

Caddoo, W. (2000, August). Personal communication.

Caplan, G. (1964). *Principles of preventive psychiatry.* New York: Basic Books.

Capra, F. (1996). *The web of life.* New York: Anchor Books.

Carr, J. L. (2005, February). *American College Health Association campus violence white paper.* Baltimore, MD: American College Health Association.

Castro, F., Barrera, M., Jr., & Martinez, C., Jr. (2004). The cultural adaptation of prevention interventions: Resolving tensions between fidelity and fit. *Prevention Science, 5,* 41–45.

Center for the Study and Prevention of Violence. (1996). Retrieved May 10, 2008, from http://www.colorado.edu/cspv/

Center for the Study and Prevention of Violence. (2002–2004). *Blueprints for violence prevention.* Retrieved September 24, 2008, from http://www.colorado.edu/cspv/blueprints/

Centers for Disease Control and Prevention. (2005). *Child maltreatment prevention.* Retrieved November 6, 2008, from http://www.cdc.gov/ncipc/dvp/CMP/CMP-conque.htm

CFED/REAL. (1993). *Team evaluation.* Retrieved April 16, 2008, from www.cfed.org/image

Chronister, K., McWhirter, B., & Kerewsky, S. (2004). Counseling and ecological prevention practice. In R. Conyne & E. Cook (Eds.), *Ecological counseling: An innovative approach to conceptualizing person–environment interaction* (pp. 315–338). Alexandria, VA: American Counseling Association.

Clancy, C. (2008). *Navigating the health care system: Advice columns from Dr. Carolyn Clancy.* Retrieved June 8, 2008, from http://www.ahrq.gov/consumer/cc/cc050608.htm

Coie, J., Watt, N., West, S., Hawkins, J., Asarnow, J., Markman, H., et al. (1993). The science of prevention: A conceptual framework and some directions for a national research program. *American Psychologist, 48,* 1013–1022.

Collaborative for Academic, Social, and Emotional Learning. (2003). *Safe and sound: An educational leader's guide to evidence-based social and emotional learning (SEL) programs.* Chicago: Author.

Collins, L., Murphy, S., & Bierman, K. (2004). A conceptual framework for adaptive preventive interventions. *Prevention Science, 5,* 185–196.

Collins, J., & Porras, J. (1997). Organizational vision and visionary organizations. *California Management Review, 34,* 234–260.

Conyne, R. (1975). Mapping for counselor action. *Personnel & Guidance Journal, 54,* 150–155.

Conyne, R. (1978). An analysis of student-environment mismatches. *Journal of College Student Personnel, 19,* 461–465.

Conyne, R. (1989). *How personal growth and task groups work.* Newbury Park, CA: Sage.

Conyne, R. (1999). *Failures in group work: How we can learn from our mistakes.* Thousand Oaks, CA: Sage.

Conyne, R. (2000). Prevention in counseling psychology: At long last, has the time now come? *The Counseling Psychologist, 28,* 838–844.

Conyne, R. (2004). *Preventive counseling: Helping people to become empowered in systems and settings* (2nd ed.). New York: Brunner-Routledge.

Conyne, R. (2008a, March 8). What we know and need to know in prevention: Stimulating a discussion. In A. Horne (Chair), *Advances in the study of prevention.* Presented at the International Counseling Psychology Conference, Chicago.

Conyne, R. (2008b, May 9). *Ecological counseling: The case of obesity.* Keynote address at the First Annual Ecological Counseling Conference, Cincinnati, OH.

Conyne, R., & Clack, R. J. (1981). *Environmental assessment and design: A new tool for the applied behavioral scientist.* New York: Praeger.

Conyne, R., & Cook, E. (Eds.). (2004). *Ecological counseling: An innovative approach to conceptualizing person–environment interaction.* Alexandria, VA: American Counseling Association.

Conyne, R., Crowell, J., & Newmeyer, M. (2008). *Group techniques: How to use them more purposefully.* Upper Saddle River, NJ: Prentice Hall.

Conyne, R., & Hage, S. (in press). Prevention groups. In B. Erford (Ed.), *Encyclopedia of counseling.* Alexandria, VA: American Counseling Association.

Conyne, R., & Horne, A. (Eds.). (2001). The use of groups for prevention [Special issue]. *Journal for Specialists in Group Work, 26.*

Conyne, R., & Newmeyer, M. (2008, March 6). *Teaching prevention.* Invited workshop presented through the Prevention Section at the 2008 International Counseling Psychology Conference, Chicago.

Conyne, R., Newmeyer, M., Kenny, M., Romano, J., & Matthews, C. (2008). Two key strategies for teaching prevention: Specialized course and infusion. In J. O'Neil & P. Britner (Eds.), Special issue on the teaching of primary prevention. *Journal of Primary Prevention.* Online publication date September 19, 2008, pp. 375–401.

Conyne, R., Newmeyer, M., & Kitchens, B. (2007, August 17). *Teaching preventive counseling: Bringing the real world into the classroom to promote social justice.* Presented at the annual meeting of the American Psychological Association, San Francisco.

Conyne, R., Rapin, L., & Rand, J. (1997). A model for leading task groups. In H. Forester-Miller & J. Kottler (Eds.), *Issues and challenges for group practitioners* (pp. 117–132). Denver, CO: Love.

Conyne, R., & Wilson, F. R. (2000). *Recommendations of the task force for the use of groups in prevention* (Division 49 position paper). Unpublished manuscript.

Cowen, E. (2000). Community psychology and routes to psychological wellness. In J. Rappaport & E. Seidman (Eds.), *Handbook of community psychology* (pp. 79–99). New York: Kluwer.

Craig, D. (1978). *HIP pocket guide to planning and evaluation.* Austin, TX: Learning Concepts.

Craik, K. (1991). The lived day of an individual: A person–environment perspective. In W. B. Walsh, K. Craik, & R. Price (Eds.), *Person–environment psychology: New directions and perspectives* (pp. 233–266). Mahwah, NJ: Lawrence Erlbaum.

Crane, M. (2008, October 22). Suicides up for middle-age whites. *The Columbus Dispatch* (News Section). Retrieved October 23, 2008, from http://www.dispatch.com/live/content/local_news/stories/2008/10/22/suicide_rates.ART_ART_10–22–08_A1_2JBLUBE .html?sid=101

Crow, S. (2002). Soak up the sun. On *C'mon C'mon* [CD]. Santa Monica, CA: Interscope Records.

Croyle, W. (2007, December 10). Dropout-free school goes the extra mile to help its students. *New York Times,* reprinted in *Cincinnati Enquirer,* p. B-1.

Csikszentmihalyi, M. (1990). *Flow: The psychology of optimal experience.* New York: Harper & Row.

D'Andrea, M., & Daniels, J. (2001). RESPECTFUL counseling: An integrative multidimensional model for counselors. In D. Pope-Davis & H. Coleman (Eds.), *The intersection of race, class, and gender in multicultural counseling* (pp. 417–466). Thousand Oaks, CA: Sage.

Danish, S., & Forneris, T. (2006). Teaching life skills in schools. In M. Elias & H. Arnold (Eds.), *The educator's guide to emotional intelligence and academic achievement: Social-emotional learning in the classroom* (pp. 188–197). Thousand Oaks, CA: Corwin.

Davidson, M., Waldo, M., & Adams, E. (2006). Promoting social justice through prevention interventions. In R. Toporek, L. Gerstein, N. Fouad, G. Roysircar, & T. Israel (Eds.), *Handbook for social justice in counseling psychology: Leadership, vision, and action* (pp. 117–129). Thousand Oaks, CA: Sage.

DeAngelis, T. (1994, June). Government should support realistic prevention projects. *APA Monitor,* pp. 32–33.

DeAngelis, T. (2008). Protecting our children. *Monitor on Psychology, 39,* 45–47.

DeLucia-Waack, J. (2006). *Leading psychoeducational groups for children and adolescents.* Thousand Oaks, CA: Sage.

Department of Health and Human Services. (2001). *Surgeon General launches effort to develop action plan to combat overweight, obesity.* Retrieved May 20, 2001, from http://www.surgeongeneral.gov/obesityprevention/index.html

Devaney, E., O'Brien, M. U., Resnik, H., Keister, S., & Weissberg, R. (2006). *Sustainable schoolwide social and emotional learning (SEL): Implementation guide and toolkit.* Chicago: CASEL.

Development Services Group. (n.d.). *Useful websites.* Retrieved September 26, 2008, from www.dsgonline.com

Division of Adolescent and School Health. (1995). *Youth risk behavior surveillance: National College Health Risk Behavior Survey—United States.* National Center for Chronic Disease Prevention and Health Promotion, Division of Adolescent and School Health. Retrieved June 10, 2008, from http://www.surgeongeneral.gov/news/pressreleases/obesitypressrelease.htm

Dodge, K. (2008). Framing public policy and prevention of chronic violence in American youths. *American Psychologist, 63,* 573–590.

Dryfoos, J. (1997). The prevalence of problem behaviors: Implications for programs. In R. Weissberg, T. Gullotta, R. Hampton, B. Ryan, & G. Adams (Eds.), *Healthy children 2010: Enhancing children's wellness* (pp. 17–46). Thousand Oaks, CA: Sage.

Dryfoos, J. G. (2000). *Evaluations of community schools: Findings to date.* Hastings-on-Hudson, NY: Coalition for Community Schools.

Duch, B., Groh, E., & Allen, D. E. (2001). *The power of problem-based learning.* Sterling, VA: Stylus Publishing.

Duckworth, B., Peterson, C., Matthews, M., & Kelly, D. (2007). Grit: Perseverance and passion for long-term goals. *Journal of Personality and Social Psychology, 92,* 1087–1101.

Dumka, L., Mauricio, A.-M., & Gonzales, N. (2007). Research partnerships with schools to implement prevention programs for Mexican origin families. *Journal of Primary Prevention, 28,* 403–420.

Durlak, J. (2003). Effective prevention and health promotion programming. In T. Gullotta & M. Bloom (Eds.), *Encyclopedia of primary prevention and health promotion* (pp. 61–69). New York: Kluwer.

Durlak, J., & Wells, A. (1997). Primary prevention programs for children and adolescents: A meta-analytic review. *American Journal of Community Psychology, 25,* 115–152.

Dusenbury, L., & Hansen, W. (2004). Pursuing the course from research to practice. *Prevention Science, 5,* 55–59.

Editorial: An early date with the dentist. (2008, March 1). *Cincinnati Enquirer,* Community Forum section, p. C-6.

Editorial: Following a new path to fitness. (2008, January 24). *Cincinnati Enquirer,* p. C-6.

Edwards, R., Jumper-Thurman, B., Plested, B., Oetting, E., & Swanson, L. (2000). Community readiness: Research to practice. *Journal of Community Psychology, 28,* 291–307.

Elden, M., & Levin, M. (1991). Cogenerative learning: Bringing participation into action research. In W. F. Whyte (Ed.), *Participatory action research* (pp. 127–142). Newbury Park, CA: Sage.

Elias, M. (1995). Primary prevention as health and social competence promotion. *Journal of Primary Prevention, 16,* 5–24.

Elias, M., & Branden, L. (1988). Primary prevention of behavioral and emotional problems in school-age populations. *School Psychology Review, 17,* 581–592.

Elias, M. J., Gager, P., & Leon, S. (1997). Spreading a warm blanket of prevention over all children: Guidelines for selecting substance abuse and related prevention curricula for use in the schools. *Journal of Primary Prevention, 18,* 41–69.

Elias, M., O'Brien, M. U., & Weissberg, R. (2006). *Transformative leadership for social-emotional learning: Principal leadership.* Bethesda, MD: National Association of Secondary School Principals, Student Services.

Elliott, D., & Mihalic, S. (2004). Issues in disseminating and replicating effective prevention programs. *Prevention Science, 5,* 47–53.

Erickson, E. (1986). *Vital involvement in old age.* New York: Norton.

Ettin, M., Heiman, M., & Kopel, S. (1988). Group building: Developing protocols for psychoeducational groups. *Group, 12,* 205–225.

Fenichel, M. (1989). Spokeswoman for our time. *Psychology Today, 23,* 71.

Finn, J., & Jacobson, M. (2003). *Just practice: A social justice approach to social work.* Peosta, IA: eddie bowers publishing.

Fleming, J., & Courtney, B. (1984). The dimensionality of self-esteem: II. Hierarchical facet model for revised measurement scales. *Journey of Personality and Social Psychology, 46,* 404–421.

Flexner, S. B. (Ed.). (1993). *The Random House Dictionary of the English Language.* New York: Random House.

Frankl, V. (1959). *Man's search for meaning.* Boston: Beacon Press.

Frederickson, B. (1998). What good are positive emotions? *Review of General Psychology, 2,* 300–319.

Fujishin, R. (2001). *Creating effective groups: The art of small group communication.* San Francisco: Acada.

Fung, J. (2008). *The wisdom of prevention.* Retrieved March 1, 2008, from http://www.youtube.com/watch?v=9NbUp8UpHHE

Glynn, R. (2008, May 18). Botched bunt clears way for one big swing. *Cincinnati Enquirer,* p. C-9.

Goldberg, N. (2008). *Dr. Niece Goldberg's complete guide to women's health.* New York: Ballantine.

Goldston, D., Molock, S. D., Whiteck, L., Murakami, J., Zayas, L., & Nagayama Hall, G. (2008). Cultural considerations in adolescent suicide prevention and psychosocial treatment. *American Psychologist, 63,* 14–31.

Good habits yield longer life, study says. (2008, January 9). *Cincinnati Enquirer,* p. A-6. Retrieved January 7, 2008, from http://medicine.plosjournals.org/

Goodman, R. (2008, May 20). Group: Kids need positives. *Cincinnati Enquirer,* pp. B-1, B-5.

Gordon, R. (1983). An operational classification of disease prevention. *Public Health Reports, 98,* 107–109.

Gottfredson, D., Fink, C., Skroban, S., & Gottfredson, G. (1997). Making prevention work. In R. Weissberg, T. Gullotta, R. Hampton, B. Ryan, & G. Adams (Eds.), *Establishing preventive services* (pp. 219–252). Thousand Oaks, CA: Sage.

Grady, D. (2008, January 21). Caffeine in pregnancy may raise miscarriage risk. *Cincinnati Enquirer,* p. A-1.

Green, L. (2007). *A resource for instructors, students, health practitioners, and researchers using the Precede-Proceed model for health program planning and evaluation.* Retrieved March 20, 2008, from http://www.lgreen.net/

Green, L., & Kreuter, M. (1999). *Health promotion planning: An educational and ecological approach* (3rd ed.). Mountain View, CA: Mayfield.

Green, L., & Ottoson, J. (2007, January). From efficacy to effectiveness to community and back: Evidence-based practice vs. practice-based evidence. In *Proceedings for clinical trials to community: The science of translating diabetes and obesity research* (pp. 15–18). Bethesda, MD: National Institutes of Health.

Greenglass, E., Schwarzer, R., & Taubert, S. (1999). *The Proactive Coping Inventory (PCI): A multidimensional research instrument.* Retrieved May 1, 2008, from http://userpage.fuberlin.de/health/greenpci.htm

Griffin, J., & Miller, E. (2007). A research practitioner's perspective on culturally-relevant prevention: Scientific and practical considerations for community-based programs. *The Counseling Psychologist, 35,* 850–859.

Grossman, J., & Tierney, J. (1998). Does mentoring work? An impact study of the Big Brothers Big Sisters program. *Evaluation Review, 22,* 403–426.

Guide to community services. (2008). Retrieved April 15, 2008, from http://www.thecommunityguide.org

Gullotta, T., & Bloom, M. (Eds.). (2003). *Encyclopedia of primary prevention and health promotion.* New York: Kluwer.

Hage, S., Romano, J., Conyne, R., Kenny, M., Matthews, C., Schwartz, J., et al. (2007). Best practice guidelines on prevention practice, research, training, and social advocacy for psychologists. *The Counseling Psychologist, 35,* 493–566.

Hawkins, J., & Catalano, R., Jr. (1992). *Preparing for the drug-free years.* San Francisco: Jossey-Bass.

Hays, P. (1996). Addressing the complexities of culture and gender in counseling. *Journal of Counseling and Development, 74,* 332–338.

Heart health. (2008, February 11). [Advertising section]. *Newsweek,* p. 8.

Heatherton, T., & Wyland, C. (2003). Assessing self-esteem. In S. Lopez & C. R. Snyder (Eds.), *Positive psychological assessment: A handbook of models and measures* (pp. 219–225). Washington, DC: American Psychological Association.

Heinlein, R. (1961). *Stranger in a strange land.* New York: Putnam.

Hingson, R., Heeren, T., Zakocs, R., Kopstein, A., & Wechsler, H. (2002). Magnitude of alcohol-related mortality and morbidity among U.S. college students ages 18–24. *Journal of Studies on Alcohol, 63,* 136–144.

Horne, A. (2005). *Bullying prevention* [Video]. Washington, DC: American Psychological Association.

Horne, A. (2008, March 8). *Advances in the study of prevention.* Program presented at the International Counseling Psychology Conference, Chicago.

Huff, R., & Kline, M. (Eds.). (1999). *Promoting health in multicultural populations: A handbook for practitioners.* Thousand Oaks, CA: Sage.

Hulse-Killacky, D., Killacky, J., & Donigian, J. (2001). *Making task groups work in your world*. Upper Saddle River, NJ: Prentice Hall.

Hunsaker, R. (2008). Social justice: An inconvenient irony. *Counseling Today, 50*(10), 21, 43.

Ilardi, S., Jacobson, J., Lehman, K., Stites, B., Karwoski, L., Stroupe, N., et al. (2007, November). *Therapeutic lifestyle change for depression: Results from a randomized controlled trial*. Presented at the annual meeting of the Association for Behavioral and Cognitive Therapy, Philadelphia.

Ilardi, S., & Karwoski, L. (2005). *The depression cure*. Unpublished book-length manuscript, University of Kansas, Lawrence.

Inner City Youth Opportunities. (n.d.). *Inner City Youth Opportunities: Education in motion*. Retrieved October 16, 2008, from http://www.icyo.us/ICYO.pdf

Institute of Medicine. (2001). *Crossing the quality chasm: A new health system for the 21st century*. Washington, DC: National Academies Press.

Israel, B., Schultz, A., Parker, E., & Becker, A. (1998). Review of community-based research: Assessing partnership approaches to improve public health. *Annual Review of Public Health, 19*, 173–202.

Jacobson, M., & Rugeley, C. (2007). Community-based participatory research: Group work for social justice and community change. *The Journal of Primary Prevention, 30*, 21–39.

Joyce, J. (1961). *Ulysses* (Corrected and reset). New York: Vantage International.

Kaczmarek, P. (2006). Counseling psychology and strengths-based counseling: A promise yet to materialize. *The Counseling Psychologist, 34*, 90–95.

Kagawa-Singer, M., & Chung, R. (1994). A paradigm for culturally based care in ethnic minority populations. *Journal of Community Psychology, 22*, 192–208.

Karjane, H., Fisher, B., & Cullen, F. (2002). *Campus sexual assault: How America's institutions of higher education respond* (Final Report, NIJ Grant #1999-WA-VX-008). Newton, MA: Education Development Center. Retrieved April 11, 2008, from http://www.uc.edu/criminaljustice/ProjectReports/Sexual_Assault.pdf

Kasambira, K., & Edwards, L. (2000). Counseling and human ecology: A conceptual framework for counselor educators. In *Proceedings of the Eighth International Counseling Conference: Counseling and human ecology* (pp. 43–52), San Jose, Costa Rica.

Kazdin, A. (2008). Evidence-based treatment and practice: New opportunities to bridge clinical research and practice, enhance the knowledge base, and improve patient care. *American Psychologist, 63*, 146–159.

Keefe, B. (2008, May 16). Woman indicted in online bullying. *Cincinnati Enquirer*, p. A-2.

Kelly, J. (2004). Popular opinion leaders and HIV prevention peer education: Resolving discrepant findings, and implications for the development of effective community programmes. *AIDS Care, 16*, 139–150.

Kelly, J., & Hess, R. (Eds.). (1987). *The ecology of prevention: Illustrating mental health consultation*. New York: Haworth.

Kenny, M., Horne, A., Orpinas, P., & Reese, L. (Eds.). (2009). *Realizing social justice: The challenge of preventive interventions*. Washington, DC: American Psychological Association.

Kenny, M., & Romano, J. (2009). Promoting positive development and social justice through prevention: A legacy to the future. In M. Kenny, A. Horne, P. Orpinas, & L. Reese (Eds.), *Realizing social justice: The challenge of preventive interventions* (pp. 17–36). Washington, DC: American Psychological Association.

Kettner, P., Moroney, R., & Martin, L. (2008). *Designing and managing programs: An effectiveness-based approach* (3rd ed.). Thousand Oaks, CA: Sage.

Keyes, C. (2007). Promoting and protecting mental health as flourishing: A complementary strategy for improving national mental health. *American Psychologist, 62*, 95–108.

Keyes, C., & Lopez, S. (2002). Toward a science of mental health: Positive directions in diagnosis and treatment. In C. R. Snyder & S. Lopez (Eds.), *The handbook of positive psychology* (pp. 45–59). New York: Oxford University Press.

Khaw, K.-T., Wareham, N., Bingham, S., Welch, A., Luben, R., & Day, N. (2007). Combined impact of health behaviors and mortality in men and women: The EPIC-Norfolk Prospective Population Study. *PloS Medicine, 5*(1), e12doi:10.1371/journal.pmed.0050012.

Kilmartin, C. (2001). *Sexual assault in context: Teaching college men about gender.* Holmes Beach, FL: Learning Publications.

King, A., Friedman, R., Marcus, B., Castro, C., Napolitano, M., Ahn, D., et al. (2007). Ongoing physical activity advice by humans versus computers: The Community Health Advice by Telephone (CHAT) trial. *Health Psychology, 26,* 718–727.

Kormanski, C. (1999). *The team: Explorations in group process.* Denver, CO: Love.

Kumpfer, K., Alvarado, R., Smith, P., & Bellamy, N. (2002). Cultural sensitivity and adaptation in family based interventions. *Prevention Science, 3,* 241–246.

Lancashire, I. (2008). *Thyrsis: A monody, to commemorate the author's friend, Arthur Hugh Clough.* Toronto, Canada: University of Toronto, Department of English. Retrieved November 19, 2008, from http://rpo.library.utoronto.ca/poem/109.html

Layton, M. J. (2008, October 15). Live to see another day. *The Record* [Online edition]. Retrieved October 18, 2008, from www.NorthJersey.com

Lee, C. (2007). *Counseling for social justice* (2nd ed.). Alexandria, VA: American Counseling Association.

Leffert, N., Benson, P., Scales, P., Sharma, A., Drake, D., & Blyth, D. (1998). Developmental assets: Measurement and prediction of risk behaviors among adolescents. *Applied Developmental Science, 2,* 209–230.

Lewin, K. (1936). *Principles of topological psychology.* New York: McGraw-Hill.

Lewin, K. (1943). Defining the "field at a given time." *Psychological Review, 50,* 292–310.

Lewis, J., Arnold, M., House, R., & Toporek, R. (2002). *Advocacy competencies: Task force on advocacy competency.* Alexandria, VA: American Counseling Association.

Lewis, C., Battistich, V., & Schaps, E. (1990). School-based primary prevention: What is an effective program? *New Directions for Child Development, 50,* 35–59.

Little, B., & Madigan, R. (1994, August). *Motivation in work teams: A test of the construct of collective efficacy.* Paper presented at the annual meeting of the Academy of Management, Houston, TX.

Lopez, S., Janowski, K., & Wells, K. (2005). *Developing strengths in college students: Exploring programs, contents, theories, and research.* Unpublished manuscript, University of Kansas, Lawrence (cited in Snyder & Lopez, 2007).

Lopez, S., & Snyder, C. (Eds.). (2003). *Positive psychological assessment: A handbook of models and measures.* Washington, DC: American Psychological Association.

Lynch, J. (1977). *The broken heart: Medical consequences of loneliness.* Baltimore, MD: Bancroft Press.

Lynch, J. (2000). *A cry unheard: New insights into the medical consequences of loneliness.* Baltimore, MD: Bancroft Press.

Lyubomirsky, S., Sousa, L., & Dickerhoof, R. (2006). The costs and benefits of writing, talking, and thinking about life's triumphs and defeats. *Journal of Personality and Social Psychology, 90,* 692–708.

Masten, A. (2001). Ordinary magic: Resilience processes in development. *American Psychologist, 56,* 227–238.

Masten, A., & Reed, M.-G. (2002). Resilience in development. In C. Snyder & S. Lopez (Eds.), *Handbook of positive psychology* (pp. 74–88). New York: Oxford University Press.

Maton, K. (2000). Making a difference: The social ecology of social transformation. *American Journal of Community Psychology, 28,* 25–57.

Matthews, C. (2003, August). Training for prevention competency in counseling psychology. In M. Kenny (Chair), *Competencies for prevention training in counseling psychology.* Symposium presented at the 111th Annual Convention of the American Psychological Association, Toronto, Ontario, Canada.

Matthews, C. (2004). *Counseling and prevention: How is the field doing?* Unpublished manuscript.

Maxwell, J. (2002). *Teamwork makes the dream work.* Nashville, TN: Thomas Nelson.

McFerrin, B. (1988). Don't worry, be happy. On *Simple pleasures* [CD]. New York: EMI.

McMahon, B., & Pugh, T. (1970). *Epidemiology: Principles and methods.* Boston, MA: Little, Brown and Company.

McWhirter, E. (1994). *Counseling for empowerment.* Alexandria, VA: American Counseling Association.

McWhirter, J., McWhirter, B., McWhirter, A.,& McWhirter, E. (1995). Youth at risk: Another point of view. *Journal of Counseling & Development, 73,* 567–569.

Mercer, J., & Arlen, H. (1944). Accentuate the positive. On *Here come the waves* [Film musical score]. New York: MPL Communications. Retrieved November 1, 2008, from www.johnnymercer.com

Mercy, J., Krug, E., Dahlberg, L., & Zwi, A. (2003). Violence and health: The United States in a global perspective. *American Journal of Public Health, 92,* 256–261.

Mertens, D. (2008). *Transformative research and evaluation.* New York: Guilford Press.

Meyers, L. (2008). Art imitating live: An innovative program at the University of Texas uses theater to fight relationship violence. *Monitor on Psychology, 39,* 44–46.

Moore, M., & Delworth, U. (1976). *Training manual for student service program development.* Boulder, CO: WICHE.

Morrill, W., Oetting, E., & Hurst, J. (1974). Dimensions of counselor functioning. *Personnel and Guidance Journal, 52,* 354–359.

Morrissey, E., Wandersman, A., Seybolt, D., Nation, M., Crusto, C., & Davino, K. (1997). Toward a framework for bridging the gap between science and practice in prevention: A focus on evaluator and practitioner perspectives. *Evaluation and Program Planning, 20,* 367–377.

Mracek, K. (2008, April 16). Table manners: Helpful hints can get you through business meals. *Cincinnati Enquirer,* p. E-2.

Mrazek, P., & Haggerty, R. (Eds.). (1994). *Reducing risks for mental disorders: Frontiers for preventive intervention.* Washington, DC: National Academy Press.

Nation, M., Crusto, C., Wandersman, A., Kumpfer, K., Seybolt, D., Morrissey-Kane, E., et al. (2003). What works in prevention: Principles of effective prevention programs. *American Psychologist, 58,* 449–456.

National Center for Education Statistics. (2003–2004). *Fast facts.* Washington, DC: U.S. Department of Education, Institute of Educational Sciences. Retrieved October 20, 2008, from http://nces.ed.gov/fastfacts/display.asp?id=60

National Institute of Justice & Centers for Disease Control. (2000, July 13). *Extent, nature, and consequences of intimate partner violence.* Washington, DC: Department of Justice.

National registry of evidence-based programs and practices. (n.d.). Retrieved March 16, 2008, from http://www.nrepp.samhsa.gov

National Youth Anti-Drug Media Campaign. (2008). *Parents: The anti-drug.* Retrieved March 11, 2008, from http://theantidrug.com/indes.asp?id=household2

Neufeld, J., Rasmussen, H., Lopez, S., Ryder, J., Magyar-Moe, J., Ford, A., et al. (2006). The engagement model of person–environment interaction. *The Counseling Psychologist, 34,* 245–259.

New Economic Foundation. (2006). *The Happy Planet Index: An index of human well-being and environmental impact.* Retrieved October 13, 2008, from http://www.happy planetindex.org/about.htm

Norcross, J. (Ed.). (2002). *Psychotherapy relationships that work: Therapist contributions and responsiveness to patient needs.* New York: Oxford University Press.

Novotney, A. (2008). The happiness diet. *Monitor on Psychology, 39,* 24–25.

Oetting, E., Donnermeyer, J., Plested, B., Edwards, R., Kelly, K., & Beauvais, F. (1995). Assessing community readiness for prevention. *International Journal of Addictions, 30,* 659–683.

O'Farrell, P. (2007, December 4). Depressed mothers' kids are injury risk. *Cincinnati Enquirer,* pp. B-1, B-5.

Okamoto, S., LeCroy, C. W., Tann, S., Rayle, A., Kulis, S., Dustman, P., et al. (2006). The implications of ecologically based assessment for primary prevention with indigenous youth populations. *Journal of Primary Prevention, 27,* 155–170.

O'Keefe, A. (2007, August 27). *Scaling the heights: The Simon Bolivar Youth Orchestra of Venezuela.* Retrieved October 15, 2008, from http://axisolflogic.com/artman/publish/article_25164.shtml

O'Neil, J., & Britner, P. (Eds.). (in press). The teaching of primary prevention [Special issue]. *Journal of Primary Prevention.*

Pascal, G. (1959). *Behavioral change in the clinic.* New York: Grune and Stratton.

Patton, M. Q. (1997). *Utilization-focused evaluation* (3rd ed.). Thousand Oaks, CA: Sage.

Peale, C. (2008, April 20). Higher education: Colleges now try to ID, help troubled students. *Cincinnati Enquirer,* p. B-2.

Pentz, M. (2004). Form follows function: Designs for prevention effectiveness and diffusion research. *Prevention Science, 5,* 23–29.

Pentz, M., Mihalic, S., & Grotpeter, J. (1998). *Blueprints for violence prevention, Book one: The Midwestern Prevention Project.* Boulder, CO: Center for the Study and Prevention of Violence. Retrieved September 24, 2008, from http://www.colorado.edu/cspv/blueprints/modelprograms/MPP.html

Peterson, C., & Seligman, M. (Eds.). (2004). *Character strengths and virtues: A handbook and classification.* Washington, DC: American Psychological Association and Oxford University Press.

Phelan, K., Khoury, J., Atherton, H., & Kahn, R. (2007). Maternal depression, child behavior, and injury. *Injury Prevention, 13,* 403–408.

Pitts, L., Jr. (2008, May 19). We shouldn't have to "live with" an unjust justice system. *Cincinnati Enquirer,* p. B-5.

Pranke, P. (2006). *Combating violence against women.* Jamestown, ND: Jamestown College, Faculty On-Line Text. Retrieved September 22, 2008, from http://www.jc.edu/campus/centerEthics/cccOnlineText.php

Presley, C., Meilman, P., & Cashin, J. (1997). Weapon carrying and substance abuse among college students. *Journal of American College Health, 46,* 3–8.

Price, R. (1974). Etiology, the social environment, and the prevention of psychological dysfunction. In P. Insel & R. Moos (Eds.), *Health and the social environment* (pp. 287–303). Lexington, MA: Heath.

Price, R., Cowen, E., Lorion, R., & Ramos-McKay, J. (Eds.). (1988). *14 ounces of prevention: A casebook for practitioners.* Washington, DC: American Psychological Association.

Prilleltensky, I., & Nelson, G. (1997). Community psychology: Reclaiming social Justice. In D. Fox & I. Prilleltensky (Eds.), *Critical psychology: An introduction* (pp. 166–184). Thousand Oaks, CA: Sage.

Prilleltensky, I., & Nelson, G. (2002). *Doing psychology critically: Making a difference in diverse settings.* Basingstoke, England: Palgrave.

Prochaska, J., & DiClemente, C. (2005). The transtheoretical approach. In J. Norcross & M. Goldfried (Eds.), *Handbook of psychotherapy integration* (pp. 141–171). New York: Oxford University Press.

Quest Network. (2006). *Live longer, better: Longevity secrets.* Quest Network. Retrieved October 8, 2008, from http://quest.bluezones.com/live-longer-better

Radcliffe, H. (2008, July 20). *El Sistema: Changing lives through music.* Retrieved October 15, 2008, from http://www.cbsnews.com

Rappaport, J. (1972). From an address delivered for Psi Chi, University of Illinois. Cited in R. Goodyear, 1976, Counselors as community psychologists, *Personnel and Guidance Journal, 54,* 513.

Rappaport, J. (1981). In praise of paradox: A social policy of empowerment over prevention. *American Journal of Community Psychology, 9,* 1–25.

Reamer, F. (1995). *The philosophical foundations of social work.* New York: Columbia University Press.

Reese, L., & Vera, E. (2007). Major contribution—Culturally relevant prevention: The scientific and practical considerations of community-based programs. *The Counseling Psychologist, 35,* 763–778.

Reese, L., Vera, E., Simon, T., & Ikeda, R. (2000). The role of families and care-givers as risk and protective factors in preventing youth violence. *Clinical Child Family Psychology Review, 3,* 61–77.

Reese, L., Wingfield, J., & Blumenthal, D. (2009). Advancing prevention and health promotion through practical integration of prevention science and practice. In M. Kenny, A. Horne, P. Orpinas, & L. Reese (Eds.), *Realizing social justice: The challenge of preventive interventions* (pp. 37–56). Washington, DC: American Psychological Association.

Reiss, D., & Price, R. (1996). National research agenda for prevention research: The National Institute of Mental Health Report. *American Psychologist, 51,* 1109–1115.

Resnicow, K., Solar, R., Braithwaite, R., Ahluwalia, J., & Butler, J. (2000). Cultural sensitivity in substance abuse prevention. *Journal of Community Psychology, 28,* 271–290.

Riessman, F. (1965). The "helper" therapy principle. *Social Work, 10,* 27–32.

Rollnick, S., & Miller, W. R. (1995). What is motivational interviewing? *Behavioural and Cognitive Psychotherapy, 23,* 325–334.

Romano, J., & Hage, S. (2000). Major contribution: Prevention in counseling psychology. *The Counseling Psychologist, 28,* 733–763.

Ryff, C. (1989). Happiness is everything, or is it? Explorations on the meaning of psychological meaning. *Journal of Personality and Social Psychology, 57,* 1069–1081.

Sackett, D., Straus, S., Richardson, W., Rosenberg, W., & Haynes, R. (2000). Evidence-based medicine: What it is and what it isn't. *British Medical Journal, 31,* 71–72.

SAPAC: Sexual Assault Prevention and Counseling. (n.d.). Retrieved September 22, 2008, from http://www.scs.unr.edu/~sapac/101/1Welcome.html

Satir, V. (1972). *Peoplemaking.* Palo Alto, CA: Science and Behavior Books.

Savery, J. (2006). Overview of problem-based learning: Definitions and distinctions. *International Journal of Problem-Based Learning, 1,* 9–20.

Schwarz, R. (2002). *The skilled facilitator: A comprehensive resource for consultants, facilitators, manager, trainers, and coaches.* San Francisco: Jossey-Bass.

Schwarzer, R., & Knoll, N. (2003). Proactive coping: Mastering demands and searching for meaning. In S. Lopez & C. Snyder (Eds.), *Positive psychological assessment: A handbook of models and measures* (pp. 393–409). Washington, DC: American Psychological Association.

Scott, E. (2008, November 8). *Time to get happy!* (About.com stress management guide). Retrieved November 10, 2008, from http://stress.about.com/b/2008/11/08/time-to-get-happy.htm?nl=1

Seligman, M. (2002a). *Authentic happiness: Using the new positive psychology to realize your potential for lasting fulfillment.* New York: Free Press.

Seligman, M. (2002b). Positive psychology, positive prevention, and positive therapy. In C. Snyder & S. Lopez (Eds.), *Handbook of positive psychology* (pp. 3–9). New York: Oxford University Press.

Selye, H. (1974). *Stress without distress.* Philadelphia: J. B. Lippincott Co.

Sexual Assault Prevention and Counseling Program. (n.d.). *Belief 17.* Retrieved September 26, 2008, from http://www.scs.unr.edu/~sapac/101/24verbal.html

Shaker Tour Guide. (2008, November 8, 2008). *Tour of center family dwelling.* Shaker Village at Pleasant Hill, Kentucky.

Shechtman, Z. (2001). Prevention groups for angry and aggressive children. *Journal for Specialists in Group Work, 26,* 228–236.

Slonim, M. (1991). *Children, culture, and ethnicity: Evaluating and understanding the impact.* New York: Garland.

Smith, E. (2006). Major contribution: The strength-based counseling model. *The Counseling Psychologist, 34,* 13–79.

Smith, L. (2005). Psychotherapy, classism, and the poor: Conspicuous by their absence. *American Psychologist, 60,* 687–696.

Smith, L. (2008). Positioning classism within counseling psychology's social justice agenda. *The Counseling Psychologist, 36,* 895–924.

Snyder, C., & Lopez, S. (Eds.). (2002). *Handbook of positive psychology.* New York: Oxford University Press.

Snyder, C., & Lopez, S. (Eds.). (2007). *Positive psychology: The scientific and practical explorations of human strengths.* Thousand Oaks, CA: Sage.

Sommer, R. (1974). *Tight spaces: Hard architecture and how to humanize it.* Englewood Cliffs, NJ: Prentice Hall.

Steele, F. (1973). *Physical settings and organization development.* Reading, MA: Addison-Wesley.

Stein, P., & Rowe, B. (1989). *Physical anthropology* (4th ed.). New York: McGraw-Hill.

Stith, S., Pruitt, I., Dees, J., Fronce, M., Green, N., Som, A., et al. (2006). Implementing community-based prevention programming: A review of the literature. *The Journal of Primary Prevention, 27,* 599–617.

Stufflebeam, D. (2003, October 3). *The CIPP model for evaluation.* Presentation at the annual meeting of the Oregon Program Evaluators Network, Portland, OR. Retrieved March 21, 2008, from http://www.wmich.edu/evalctr/pubs/CIPP-ModelOregon10–03.pdf

Sue, D. W. (2003). *Overcoming our racism: The journey to liberation.* San Francisco: Jossey-Bass.

Sue, D. W., Arredondo, P., & McDavis, R. (1992). Multicultural counseling competencies and standards: A call to the profession. *Journal of Counseling & Development, 70,* 477–486.

Sue, D. W., Capodilupo, C., Torino, G., Bucceri, J., Holder, A., Nadal, K., et al. (2007). Racial microaggressions in everyday life: Implications for clinical practice. *American Psychologist, 62,* 271–286.

Sue, D. W., & Constantine, M. (2005). Effective multicultural consultation and organizational development. In M. Constantine & D. W. Sue (Eds.), *Strategies for building multicultural competence in mental health and educational settings* (pp. 212–226). Hoboken, NJ: Wiley.

Sue, D. W., Nadal, K., Capodilupo, C., Lin, A., Torino, G., & Rivera, D. (2008). Racial microaggressions against Black Americans: Implications for counseling. *Journal of Counseling & Development, 86,* 330–338.

Sue, S., Zane, N., & Young, K. (1994). Research on psychotherapy with culturally diverse populations. In A. Bergin & S. Garfield (Eds.), *Handbook of psychotherapy and behavior change* (4th ed., pp. 783–817). New York: Wiley.

Swensen, C., Jr. (1968). An approach to case conceptualization. In S. Stone & B. Shertzer (Eds.), *Guidance monograph series II: Counseling* (pp. 28–29). Boston: Houghton Mifflin.

Tatara, P. (2008, October 16). *The naked city.* Retrieved October 22, 2008, from http://www.tcm.com/thismonth/article.jsp?cid=72532&mainArticleId=2

Tesh, J. (2008). *Intelligence for your life.* Retrieved December 12, 2008, from www.tesh.com

The Fischbowl. (2007, September). *Did you know? 2.0.* Retrieved October 30, 2008, from http://shifthappens.wikispaces.com

Therapeutic lifestyle change: A new treatment for depression. (2005). Lawrence: University of Kansas, Psychology Department. Retrieved October 15, 2008, from www.psych.ku .edu/tlc

Thompson, S. (2008, August). Colombia, Home to efficient happiness. *Miller-McCune,* p. 7.

Tobler, N. (2000). Lessons learned. *The Journal of Primary Prevention, 20,* 261–274.

Tobler, N., Roona, M., Ochshorn, P., Marshall, D., Strexe, A., & Stackpole, K. (2000). *The Journal of Primary Prevention, 20,* 275–336.

Tobler, N., & Stratton, H. (1997). Effectiveness of school-based drug prevention programmes: A meta-analysis of the research. *Journal of Primary Prevention, 18,* 71–128.

Toporek, R., Gerstein, L., Fouad, N., Roysircar, G., & Israel, T. (Eds.). (2006). *Handbook for social justice in counseling psychology: Leadership, vision, and action.* Thousand Oaks, CA: Sage.

Travis, C. (2006). *Daily dose of positivity: Mental supplements for better health.* Retrieved October 28, 2008, from http://www.iuniverse.com

Tripodi, T., Fellin, P., & Epstein, I. (1978). *Differential social program evaluation.* Itasca, IL: Peacock.

Try it: Exercise reminders via phone. (2008, January 8). *Cincinnati Enquirer,* p. D-1.

UNESCO. (1993). *Focusing resources on effective school health.* Retrieved September 18, 2008, from http://portal.unesco.org/education

U.S. Department of Health and Human Services. (2000). *Healthy people 2010: Understanding and improving health* (2nd ed.). Washington, DC: U.S. Government Printing Office.

U.S. Department of Health and Human Services. (2001). *The Surgeon General's call to action to prevent and decrease overweight and obesity.* Rockville, MD: Author.

U.S. Environmental Protection Agency. (2008, February 20). *Indoor air facts no. 4 (revised): Sick building syndrome.* Retrieved May 15, 2008, from http://www.epa.gov/iaq/ pubs/sbs.html#

Vera, E. (2008, March 6). Commentary on the choices program. In A. Horne (Chair), *Prevention practice: A workshop on prevention application programs that have demonstrated effectiveness.* Presentation at the 2008 International Counseling Psychology Conference, Chicago.

Vera, E., Buhin, L., & Isacco, A. (2009). The role of prevention in psychology's social justice agenda. In M. Kenny, A. Horne, P. Orpinas, & L. Reese (Eds.), *Realizing social justice: The challenge of preventive interventions* (pp. 79–96). Washington, DC: American Psychological Association.

Vera, E., Caldwell, J., Clarke, M., Gonzales, R., Morgan, M., & West, M. (2007). The Choices program: Multisystemic interventions for enhancing the personal and academic effectiveness of urban adolescents of color. *The Counseling Psychologist, 35,* 779–796.

Vera, E., & Spreight, S. (2003). Multicultural competence, social justice, and counseling psychology: Expanding our roles. *The Counseling Psychologist, 31,* 253–272.

Vinokur, A., Schul, Y., Vuori, J., & Price, R. (2000). Two years after a job loss: Long term impact of the JOBS program on reemployment and mental health. *Journal of Occupational Health Psychology, 5,* 32–47.

Violence Prevention Alliance, World Health Organization. (2008). *Global campaign for violence prevention.* Retrieved September 18, 2008, from http://www.who.int/violenceprevention/approach

Waldo, M., & Schwartz, J. (2008, March 6). *Training students in evidence-based prevention: Promoting social justice in schools.* In A. Horne (Chair), Teaching prevention: A prevention section seminar at the 2008 International Counseling Psychology Conference, Chicago, Illinois.

Walsh, M., DePaul, J., & Park-Taylor, J. (in press). In M. Kenny, A. Horne, P. Orpinas, & L. Reese (Eds.), *Handbook of prevention: Promoting positive development and social justice.* Washington, DC: American Psychological Association.

Wandersman, A., & Florin, P. (2003). Community interventions and effective prevention. *American Psychologist, 58,* 441–448.

Washington, G. (1971). *Rules of civility and decent behaviour in company and conversation: A book of etiquette.* Williamsburg, VA: Beaver Press. Retrieved April 16, 2008, from http://www.history.org/Almanack/life/manners/rules2.cfm

Watson, A., Collins, R., & Collins Correia, F. (2004). Advocacy and social action in the context of ecological counseling. In R. Conyne & E. Cook (Eds.), *Ecological counseling: An innovative approach to conceptualizing person–environment interaction* (pp. 289–313). Alexandria, VA: American Counseling Association.

Weissberg, R., & Greenberg, M. (1998). School and community competence-enhancement and prevention programs. In W. Damon (Series Ed.) and I. Sigel & K. Renninger (Vol. Eds.), *Handbook of child psychology: Vol 4. Child psychology in practice* (5th ed., pp. 877–954). New York: Wiley.

Welsh-Huggins, A. (2008, January 10). *Religion today: Moved by multiple deaths, pastor orders men to see doctors.* Retrieved January 10, 2008, from http://abcnews.go.com/US/wireStory?id=4115284

Weng, X., Odouli, R., & Li, D. K. (2008). Maternal caffeine consumption during pregnancy and the risk of miscarriage: A prospective cohort study. *American Journal of Obstetrics and Gynecology, 198,* 279–281.

Werner, E., & Smith, R. (1982). *Vulnerable but invincible: A study of resilient children.* New York: McGraw-Hill.

Werner, E., & Smith, R. (1992). *Overcoming the odds: High-risk children from birth to adulthood.* Ithaca, NY: Cornell University Press.

Wessels, J. (2008). Looking for help that helps. *Cincinnati City Beat* (Voices Section), *14,* p. 5.

White Bison. (2007). *Fathers of tradition.* Retrieved March 19, 2008, from www.whitebison.org

Wilkinson, H. (2007, December 10). Van would help VA reach vets. *Cincinnati Enquirer,* pp. B-1, B-5.

Wolfe, T. (1979). *The right stuff.* New York: Farrar, Straus, & Giroux. Retrieved April 10, 2008, from www.aarpmagazine.org/lifestyle

World Health Organization. (2002). *World report on violence and health.* Geneva, Switzerland: Author.

World Health Organization. (2004). *Preventing violence: A guide to implementing the recommendations of the world report on violence and health.* Geneva, Switzerland: Author. Retrieved September 20, 2008, from http://whqlibdoc.who.int/publications/2004/9241592079.pdf

Yee, D. (2007, December 9). Some airports offer flu shots at the gate. *Cincinnati Enquirer,* p. A-20.

Zaza, S., Briss, P., & Harris, K. (2005). *The guide to community preventive services: What works to promote health?* New York: Oxford University Press.

Zigler, E., Taussig, C., & Black, K. (1992). Early childhood intervention: A promising preventative for juvenile delinquency. *American Psychologist, 8,* 997–1006.

Author Index

Abrieu, J. A., 31
Adams, E., xi, 28
Agency for Healthcare Research and Quality, 39, 43, 71
Ahluwalia, J., 28
Ahn, D., 13
Albee, G., 4, 20–21, 26, 28, 50, 51, 177–178
Allen, D. E., 106
Alvarado, R., 40
American Academy of Periodontology, 7
American College Health Association, 155, 157
American Counseling Association, 70, 81
American Psychological Association (APA), 15–17, 42, 53, 70, 93
Anderson, N., 16
Andress, S., 69
Arlen, H., 63
Arnold, M., 25, 148
Arredondo, P., 70, 80
Asarnow, J., 35
Aspinall, L., 54
Association for Specialists in Group Work, 70
Atherton, H., 14

Baker, E., 35
Ballard, D., 111, 112
Bandura, A., 65, 68, 142, 145–146
Barrera, M., Jr., 40
Battistich, V., 38
Baum, K., 156
Baumeister, R., 55, 139
Baye, B., 89
Beauvais, F., 39
Becker, A., 92
Belch, J., 12
Bellamy, N., 40
Bemak, F., 71
Benson, P., 70

Berman, S., 41
Bierman, K., 40
Biglan, A., 81
Bingham, S., 13
Black, K., 35
Bloom, L., 5
Bloom, M., 26, 51, 146
Blumenthal, D., 36, 40
Blyth, D., 70
Boal, A., 163
Boden, J., 55
Boone, P., 10
Botvin, E., 35
Botvin, G., 35, 47, 55, 144
Braithwaite, R., 28
Brand, E., 41
Branden, L., 50
Branden, N., 139
Brim, O., 64
Briss, P., 40
Britner, P., xiii
Bronfenbrenner, U., 57, 79, 147
Brown, N., 41
Bruvold, W., 42
Bruzzese, A., 11
Buettner, D., 13
Buhin, L., 54, 70
Butler, J., 28
Byrd, T., 41, 43

Caddoo, W., 8, 144
Caldwell, J., 29, 82, 92
Campbell, I., 12
Caplan, G., 20
Capodilupo, C., 5
Capra, E., 148
Carnine, D., 81
Carr, J. L., 156, 157
Cashin, J., 156

Subject Index

About the Author

Robert K. Conyne, PhD, professor emeritus from the University of Cincinnati, is a licensed psychologist, clinical counselor, and Fellow of the Association for Specialists in Group Work (ASGW) and the American Psychological Association and three of its divisions. He has 36 years of professional experience as a university professor, department head, and program director, and as a psychologist and counselor. He has provided consultation and training over decades both within the United States and within several international contexts, including frequent assignments in China. Current work finds him volunteering as an American Red Cross disaster mental health specialist and serving as a military family life consultant. Bob has received many awards, including the Eminent Career Award from the ASGW; the Lifetime Achievement Award in Prevention, Society of Counseling Psychology of the APA; the Distinguished Alumni Award of Distinction from Purdue University; and designation as a Soros International Scholar providing service in Kyrgyzstan to the American University of Central Asia. He is the 2009 president of the APA's Division of Group Psychology and Group Psychotherapy. With over 200 scholarly publications and presentations, including 10 books in his areas of expertise (group work, prevention, and ecological counseling), along with broad international consultation in these areas, Bob is recognized as an expert in working with people and systems and across cultures. With colleague (and wife) Lynn S. Rapin, PhD, he also helps people plan and prepare psychologically for their upcoming retirement, using the holistic approach they developed, "Charting Your Personal Future." This new book on prevention program development builds on his basic text, *Preventive Counseling* (2004). His most recent offering is *Group Techniques: How to Use Them More Meaningfully* (2008, with former students Jeri Crowell and Mark Newmeyer), which demonstrates how to help group members by using an ecological orientation. When not working, Bob and Lynn—as often as possible with their children, Suzanne and Zack, who are now grown—can be found enjoying life at their northern Ontario cottage with their dog, Lucy.

Supporting researchers for more than 40 years

Research methods have always been at the core of SAGE's publishing program. Founder Sara Miller McCune published SAGE's first methods book, *Public Policy Evaluation*, in 1970. Soon after, she launched the *Quantitative Applications in the Social Sciences* series—affectionately known as the "little green books."

Always at the forefront of developing and supporting new approaches in methods, SAGE published early groundbreaking texts and journals in the fields of qualitative methods and evaluation.

Today, more than 40 years and two million little green books later, SAGE continues to push the boundaries with a growing list of more than 1,200 research methods books, journals, and reference works across the social, behavioral, and health sciences. Its imprints—Pine Forge Press, home of innovative textbooks in sociology, and Corwin, publisher of PreK–12 resources for teachers and administrators—broaden SAGE's range of offerings in methods. SAGE further extended its impact in 2008 when it acquired CQ Press and its best-selling and highly respected political science research methods list.

From qualitative, quantitative, and mixed methods to evaluation, SAGE is the essential resource for academics and practitioners looking for the latest methods by leading scholars.

For more information, visit **www.sagepub.com**.

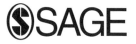